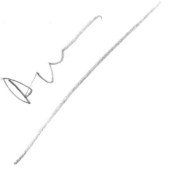

MIGHTY FLOWER

HOW CANNABIS SAVED MY SON

DR. ANNABELLE
MANALO-MORGAN, PhD.
SCIENTIST, INNOVATOR AND MOTHER

MIGHTY
FLOWER

HOW CANNABIS SAVED MY SON

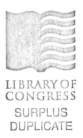

ForbesBooks

Published by ForbesBooks, Charleston, South Carolina.
Member of Advantage Media Group.

ForbesBooks is a registered trademark, and the ForbesBooks colophon is a trademark of Forbes Media, LLC.

Printed in the United States of America.

10 9 8 7 6 5 4 3 2 1

ISBN: 978-1-95086-300-6 (Hardcover)
ISBN: 978-1-95588-465-5 (eBook)

LCCN: 2022904146

Cover design by Carly Blake.
Layout design by Mary Hamilton.

This custom publication is intended to provide accurate information and the opinions of the author in regard to the subject matter covered. It is sold with the understanding that the publisher, Advantage|ForbesBooks, is not engaged in rendering legal, financial, or professional services of any kind. If legal advice or other expert assistance is required, the reader is advised to seek the services of a competent professional.

Since 1917, Forbes has remained steadfast in its mission to serve as the defining voice of entrepreneurial capitalism. ForbesBooks, launched in 2016 through a partnership with Advantage Media Group, furthers that aim by helping business and thought leaders bring their stories, passion, and knowledge to the forefront in custom books. Opinions expressed by ForbesBooks authors are their own. To be considered for publication, please visit **www.forbesbooks.com**.

For my husband Gramps and my children Aaliyah, Braylon, Macario, Yazid, and Haris ... the lights to my fire and the foundation for creating my life's story.

CONTENTS

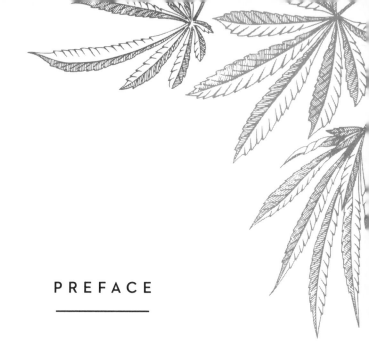

PREFACE

This book is for the young, aspiring student of life. One who shapes their dreams around personal drive and a belief that they can make a positive impact and effect change. One who wants to lead based on truth and a lack of fear in their mind. This book is a story of how, if you are open to the dynamic shifts of life, you will learn vital lessons, discover the unimaginable, make an impact, and witness miracles. This is a story about all that is wrong with our medical industry—and all that is right. This book is meant to give you a sense of where the cannabis industry is in 2022, how it came to be here, where it's headed, and how—along with modern medicine—we are in a novel place in time. Some may even call it a revolutionary place in time.

I've balanced multiple roles in life thus far—I've been a basketball player, a mother, a wife, a scientist, an entrepreneur, a healer. At my core, however, I've come to see myself as a revolutionary. That is not what I necessarily aspired to be as a young eleven-year-old girl growing up in Saskatchewan, Canada, but my experiences shaped me in ways I could never have expected—and instead of defining myself against them, I learned from them and grew strong from being able to hold all the disparate pieces of my own life's puzzle in my heart. As Walt Whitman once said, we are large—and we contain multitudes. As long as we believe in our own capabilities, we will find what life's guiding us toward. If we zoom out the lens, we can find a fluency in all the chapters of our lives—and we can begin to see the thread of purpose that binds those chapters together. Being a revolutionary simply requires recognizing that thread and putting it to good use in changing the world.

"Mighty Flower" defines me. It defines the life circumstances that have shaped me and helped me grow, and it defines my strength to not just overcome the challenges, but to incorporate them into my very substance—and to bloom. At the same time, Mighty Flower defines the cannabis plant that this book is all about—a plant that has so much power and so much potential. It's time to let cannabis bloom into everything it could be.

Annabelle Manalo, PhD, 2022

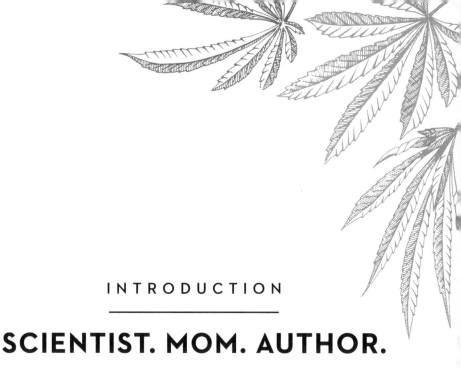

SCIENTIST. MOM. AUTHOR.

O ur bodies are amazing feats of nature. The way a single cell, or a cluster of cells, can impact other biological processes can seem random, but in fact, there's often a dynamic system at play. One element impacts another. Problems can be isolated, and yet that isolation occurs in a larger context. Processes play off one another. There's a method to the madness.

Studying problems at the microscopic level is crucial to my work as a cellular biologist and my field of disease research. And yet, so much of what we could discover about our biology—and our humanity—is only visible once we zoom out the lens.

Nothing exists in a vacuum. While uniformity and regularity may be determined by the laws of physics and biology, the fate of specific human bodies and minds are far from predictable. The reason is simple: those bodies are sentient. They can think and communicate.

They can understand language. And they exist within time and space, within cultures, civilizations, and eras.

Humans have studied their inner bodily workings for millennia. The scientific revolution, the advent of the scientific method, and the invention of the microscope are all milestones that have taken place within the last five hundred years. The history of modern medicine began just two centuries ago. With each new era of discovery, our collective knowledge and understanding of the way the world works shifts.

Old ideas are replaced and updated, and in many cases, looked upon by new generations with a sense of embarrassment or with one eyebrow raised. Ancient Egyptians believed disease was caused by supernatural powers and that the heart played an outsize role in bodily ailments.[1] Modern science proves much of Egyptian thought on diagnosis incorrect. And yet as early as 1500 BCE, this civilization had developed some healing remedies that weren't based on magic but in the natural composition of substances within their reach. They used honey as a natural antiseptic, they treated burns with aloe,[2] and they were already using opioids as painkillers and cannabis as a narcotic. Ancient Egyptian physicians described depression and dementia as physical as well as mental illnesses, born of the heart.[3] Entire generations of physicians passed before the scientific community acknowledged what the Egyptians clearly understood: that the mind–body

1   Justin Barr, "Vascular medicine and surgery in ancient Egypt," *Journal of Vascular Surgery* 60, no. 1 (July 2014): 260–263, https://www.sciencedirect.com/science/article/pii/S0741521414008659.

2   N. H. Aboelsoud, "Herbal medicine in ancient Egypt," *Journal of Medicinal Plants Research* 42, no. 2 (January 18, 2010): 62–86, https://academicjournals.org/journal/JMPR/article-full-text-pdf/F90544714963.

3   Rami Bou Khalil and Sami Richa, "When Affective Disorders Were Considered to Emanate from the Heart: The Ebers Papyrus," *American Journal of Psychiatry* 171, no. 3 (March 2014): 275, https://ajp.psychiatryonline.org/doi/pdfplus/10.1176/appi.ajp.2013.13070860.

connection is real and that mental afflictions nearly always have a biological component. That component is not the heart but the brain—and yet does this misidentification on the part of Egyptian physicians render their entire body of thought irrelevant? After all, we are internally interconnected. We don't always understand where the root of the problem comes from.

It's human nature to focus on what's in front of us. But just as a cell exists within a body that exists within a time and place, so, too, does our current scientific thought and approach.

Civilizations across the globe have relied on natural remedies to biological problems for thousands of years. And those remedies were so effective, entire schools of thought were built around them, from Chinese medicine to Ayurvedic medicine and many cultures of healing in between. The scientific community now has tools available to us that the earliest practitioners of those ancient traditions could have never dreamed of. I know firsthand what our labs are capable of

> Just as a cell exists within a body that exists within a time and place, so, too, does our current scientific thought and approach.

creating. And yet our practice of science has so far focused only on the new and has neglected to learn from those traditions, let alone integrate them into a holistic school of thought.

The prescription medication we can create in the lab has changed the world. But what are we missing? What's behind the curtain—and why aren't we collectively jumping at the chance to peek inside?

MACARIO: MY BLESSING

In 2016, I gave birth to a beautiful baby boy. My husband, Gramps Morgan, and I named him Macario. The name is the Filipino word for "blessing," and we knew that's what he would be to us. We loved him from the second we saw him. It's a special thing to be joined together by parenthood—and when I look back on the events that occurred after those first forty-eight hours, I feel blessed beyond belief that it was Gramps who was by my side the whole time. It was Gramps who first saw Macario, just two days old, foaming at the mouth, seizing, and twitching.

We rushed Macario to the hospital and were told our son had suffered from both a stroke and uncontrollable seizures. Over the next few weeks, those seizures would begin to occur up to two hundred times a day. These weeks were made up of moments that every parent dreads. Times like this are supposed to be relegated to the world of nightmares, but we couldn't wake ourselves up. Every drug regimen was attempted before we realized that the seizures would not stop and could soon take over the rest of his brain.

We were left with allowing the neurosurgery team to perform a significant brain surgery that resected 38 percent of Macario's brain. We understood that Macario would likely never speak normally, would have limited movement, and was looking at a future defined by challenges none of us could fully predict. He was on so many different prescriptions that he was nearly unresponsive. Strangers would tell me he behaved so well, like an angel. They didn't realize the reason he wasn't crying and fussing was because he was continually under the fog of medication.

After his surgery, I did what any mother would do—I desperately searched for any possible remedy or cure or aid that could help in

Macario's recovery and give him a better chance at life. And because I am a scientist by trade, I translated my desperation into invention. So many innovations are born from a time of need, underpinned by a similar desperation or life-or-death drive, and what I did in the lab for my son is no different.

In the summer of 2016, I developed the purest and most consistent form of cannabidiol, or CBD oil, that my scientific expertise would allow, with no other cannabinoids or fillers. I took my son off his heavy drug regimen and began administering my creation directly through the feeding tube protruding from his little belly.

Three years later, as I write this in 2019, Macario is now playing catch-up to his peers in preschool—and he's very nearly there. He can walk and run, he can giggle and play, and he can speak in the broken, fluttery English that defines toddlerhood. This book, and my story, begins with the blessing of Macario. This book tells the story of what bridged the huge gap between what our current scientific moment would predict for my son and what I knew was possible.

WHERE MY OWN STORY BEGINS

As a cellular biologist, my work is both methodical and spontaneous. Through my years of research and hours in the lab, I've come to understand that the road you take to reach a particular discovery or conclusion is long and winding. Certain inputs can completely change the outcome of an experiment. To be open to the multiplicity of possibilities is crucial to any good scientist's work. Life can work in a similar way—what

> To be open to the multiplicity of possibilities is crucial to any good scientist's work. Life can work in a similar way.

seems like a straight path toward the future can easily twist, turn, and sometimes throw you completely off the trail. And like a good scientist, the best way to live with the unpredictability is to simply embrace it.

I was born in Saskatchewan, Canada, a province where some of North America's first inhabitants settled, and where many of those first peoples' descendants still live. Our family was small and close, just me and my big brother Russell. Russell beat me up and teased me for having two buck teeth. My nickname was Rabbit. As most big brothers are, he was a pain in my butt, but looking back, Russell taught me to always stand my ground and that being a crybaby wasn't going to get you very far. So, we grew up in small-town Saskatchewan, but in many ways the origin of my story began halfway across the globe.

My mother was born in one of the poorest regions of the Philippines. But she was born with a gift that would change her world. She had a beautiful singing voice, and as she grew older, she'd go into town to compete in singing competitions, winning a little bit of money but making an even bigger impression. She did this for years, until one day her big break finally came: she was given the opportunity to leave the Philippines to sing for a band in Europe. After months of touring, she landed in Canada, where she met my father, a fellow Filipino who had already made his home there. They got married soon after and had two children: my brother, five years older, and me.

My mom never took her good fortune for granted. She made it her mission to provide for others the same opportunities she was blessed with. Under her guidance, our family sponsored over forty relatives from the Philippines and helped them get settled in Canada. Russell and I watched as my mother nurtured these relatives and their children, building up their confidence and helping the kids get a great education. She was like a warrior for them—but to me, she was a pioneer. The time, effort, and energy it took to create a new path for so many of her loved ones must have been incredible. But instead of being weighed down by the responsibilities she took on, she thrived. Watching what she could do when she put her mind to it—and how much she could do—was one of the greatest gifts of my childhood.

Even prior to my mother, my grandmother Lola Rose was another pioneer woman that I was able to look up to. Lola had no limits, God rest her soul. She was jumping on the trampoline with me when she was in her sixties and the only one on the dance floor at our family parties. As a young girl, that was normal to me. But as I grew up, I started to see how unique my Lola was. The memory of Lola remains dear to my heart, and I gave my first daughter, my only daughter, her name: Aaliyah Rose. I remember Lola telling stories about how poor my family in the Philippines was and how she raised thirteen children on her own. My grandfather died at a young age, but based on Lola's positive demeanor, you'd never know. My Lola never complained or spoke of her pain. She only spoke of how she found a way forward with multiple jobs and no education. And I suppose as generations pass, I can be happy that my Lola would be proud of me. That the same way she saw something special in my mom, the second oldest of all of her children, she saw something special in me.

Even before I was born, Lola came to Canada in a Saskatchewan snowstorm to be by my mom's side. My mom was the first of her family to leave the Philippines, to not be held down by circumstances, but to achieve something great and provide a platform for the rest of the family. That platform has become a foundation for me, as I'm the first of my family to receive a PhD. (Holding on to what inspires me—Aaliyah was a singer I aspired to be like. At a young age, I didn't know if I wanted to sing, play sports, bake, or become an astronaut. My mind was free. And it seems as we grow older and move further in time generationally, we lose the ability to imagine and dream.) I know my daughter, Aaliyah, will achieve something great, as the heart of my grandmother lives in her as well. I'm so grateful to be able to identify with it and guide her at such a young age.

My mother wasn't the only one who refused to limit herself based on what others thought was possible or impossible. My father, an engineer, taught me from an early age that every opportunity I could dream of was within my reach. Unlike so many parents of his generation, he didn't have a prescriptive outlook on what my future should look like. He didn't try to harness my potential or push it toward any premeditated path. Instead, like a mad scientist, he did everything he could to foster the potential itself, and as I aged, he watched it grow outward in every direction. I like to say that my dad is the reason I am who I am today. Between observing my mom and questioning my dad's love, I'd rather not choose who impacted me more. Honestly, it was the perfect formula for Dr. Annabelle.

My dad was the type of parent who never gave me praise. He was at every sporting event, he tutored me in every subject, he forced me to play the piano, and he drove me everywhere I needed to go. All while providing for my family. You see, my dad is a structural and civil engineer. He grew up believing in perfection. And it always seemed like he never demanded it from my brother, Russell. But he did from me. I remember getting praise from my peers for hitting the winning jump shot or being the only one to get over 90 percent on an exam. So many times, I'd feel like I was on top of the world! And Dad would come shut that down. Why did you throw the ball away on that play? Why did you miss a free throw? How could you get all of those questions right on your math test but get that one wrong? He always brought me back down to earth—and quick! And on my wedding day, just a few years shy of the release of this book, I realized during my father–daughter dance that the way Dad loved me, in a way that needed no words, was exactly what I needed to become me. It made me pay attention to detail. It made me take my time. It made me realize that I could always be better ... despite what everybody else was saying or portraying to me. Dad made me expect more from myself. And to this day, I always do.

A BASKETBALL DREAM, COME AND GONE

Growth isn't necessarily linear, and potential can be an unpredictable, dynamic force, capable of bursting forth in unexpected ways. It seems my father knew something essential about who I was becoming: he knew that only by following my dreams and trusting my intuition would I understand my own capacities and learn to thrive. He didn't want me to strive for perfection. Instead, encouraging me to trust in the power of my dreams and my intuition, he taught me to strive for innovation and invention—something even greater than what my imagination could dream up. He pushed me to think outside the box. And my first big dream was not just out of the box. It was out of the country.

I began my path with the singular dream of becoming a professional basketball player. As a kid in Saskatchewan, this was a big and somewhat unimaginable idea. Basketball scouts never came to our schools. It just wasn't something that happened. Thanks to the twists and turns, however, I ended up graduating early and getting recruited to play ball for Dillard University in New Orleans.

However, dreams and interests change. Sometimes, the change occurs simply as a by-product of growing up and being open and adaptive to the lessons life's trying to teach you. Other times, the course is changed because of an occurrence so big and immediate that all you thought was stable gets swept out from underneath you—and from that place, all you can do is rebuild. What's rebuilt never looks quite like what's being replaced. In 2005, Hurricane Katrina hit New Orleans and shook our world. I transferred to Eastern Kentucky University my senior year, but my dream of playing basketball got lost somewhere in the wreckage. I focused my energy on graduating, and when I was offered a chance to play basketball overseas, I turned down the opportunity to focus on a new potential that was growing in my life: a journey with my first boyfriend who had gotten drafted to the NFL. And soon, I was pregnant with my first child—Aaliyah.

PURSUING SCIENCE: ANOTHER PATH FORWARD

In the months during my pregnancy, I thought of my own mother. Kids learn from what they see, and I grew up with a mother who could do everything. Her boundless energy and passion made me feel like anything was possible just as much as my father's belief in me did. Looking up to a strong, capable mother was a core part of my experience of childhood, and I wanted to give that inspiration to my children. So, with a degree in biology and chemistry and an ongoing interest in science and medicine, I pursued an MD at Georgetown University.

Another unpredictable event changed the course of my dream of becoming a doctor—my father was diagnosed with stage IV cancer of the esophagus. As you'll read in the pages of my book, every doctor said my father would die. When he didn't, I wanted to know why—not necessarily why he, specifically, survived against all odds, but what was happening inside his body that ensured his survival, rather than his untimely death that every professional predicted.

This averted tragedy brought me closer to my higher calling. I didn't want to simply administer diagnoses to patients. I wanted to understand at a cellular level why these diagnoses occurred, what underlying mechanisms played a role, and what unexplored solutions there may be that target those mechanisms and change their expression. In my father's path to recovery, I saw the adaptive power of the body, the psychological power of belief, and the healing power of nature. My new dream was nothing short of understanding how all of these forces worked together.

Life imitates art—but it also imitates science, if we look close enough. My life led me to plenty of unpredictable outcomes. Yet when I reflect on my own story, it seems like every twist and turn was preparing me for Macario and what I was able to develop in the lab to save him, and many others since. In many ways, motherhood set my course—it showed me what was possible as a child, and I pursued higher education because I wanted to give that same inspiration to my daughter. And it was motherhood that revealed my life's true purpose. As a mother, I was willing to do anything to help my baby live and thrive. What I discovered in that desperation is what led me to write this book.

CANNABIS: LOOKING BEYOND THE LIMITS OF WHAT'S POSSIBLE

Despite an inundation of the substance in the market, most individuals still don't understand what cannabis, and in particular, cannabidiol or other molecules of the plant, can do for our health—and that includes individuals in the scientific community of which I'm a part. The industry is booming and there's money flowing in seemingly every direction outside of the lab itself. We understand the potency of cannabis as a recreational drug—but we are only on the cusp of truly understanding its medicinal powers. It's time to cast off the taboo of weed culture and approach this plant with the level of scientific rigor it deserves.

> It's time to cast off the taboo of weed culture and approach this plant with the level of scientific rigor it deserves.

Through my work developing pure cannabidiol oil in the lab during my son's time of need in 2016, I saw the huge medical potential of cannabis firsthand. And in my work since, discussing my cannabis discoveries to dozens of in-need individuals and groups around the world, I've also seen firsthand that there are countless sick individuals who don't know what they should try. This book is an attempt to get this conversation started—to share my scientific understandings and to give individuals a clearer understanding of the limitations of our scientific moment, but also the bright future ahead.

In the pages that follow, you'll find Macario's story, and how his challenges brought me to develop the best possible cannabis solution for my son that could not be found on the market. You'll learn how it helped him. But you'll also find an in-depth exploration of cannabis, both as a drug and as a taboo, and a critical analysis of what the future holds for this powerful substance, both in our country and around the globe. Cannabis is just a small part of the bigger picture. Thank you for joining me on this journey—I hope that as it unfolds in these next pages, you begin to see the untapped potential in the world of science, but also in our own bodies and minds. We are capable of great things: incredible growth, recovery, and innovation. Let this book be a testament to what we have the power to achieve once we look beyond the limits of what's possible.

The first step in any journey is believing. You can't overcome any challenge—no matter if you have the best surgeon, at the best hospital, with the best therapists and the most trusted medicine—without belief. We never treated Macario differently.

With this in mind, I would be remiss if I didn't mention the one thing that kept me strong during this entire story of mine... faith.

The truth is there is so much about my son's story that can't be scientifically explained. But the research, our abilities to try to explain such phenomena or miracles, are our best chance at definition so that we can help others. But faith played such a big role.

Why are some saved and others not? Timing. Professionals involved. Who are these people? What really drives them? Maybe these miracles are meant to remind us of our purpose—that we shouldn't only be brought together in times of tragedy. That stories bring us together. And that our brains and bodies have the ability to move in unpatterned, unplanned, and ultimately unexplained ways. And it is, in fact, the perfect patterning. So what's next?

My life represents a constant shift between technicalities and faith. In some ways, that's the core problem with the cannabis industry—it provides a hope with no direction, nothing to back it up.

So what's your mission statement? What are you chosen to offer? Who will Macario become? This book represents my awakening.

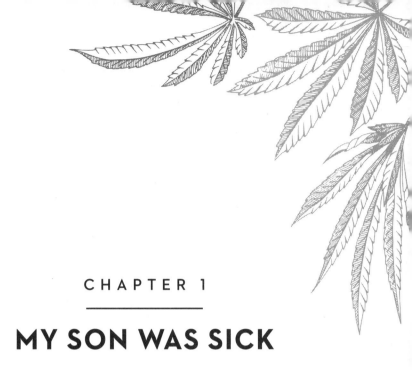

CHAPTER 1

MY SON WAS SICK

The scientific method begins with an observation. Based on an observation, you make a hypothesis. Then you design experiments to test its validity. Sometimes your experiments prove your hypothesis correct. Other times, they can reveal something far different, and often something far more exciting. Let's observe the facts.

On January 14, 2016, I gave birth to Macario. The first child of my husband Gramps Morgan and me, he was perfect. When we arrived home from the hospital, we believed the next few weeks would be a time of great joy, a period of both celebration of our new child and eager anticipation. Gramps, a talented reggae artist, had been nominated for his first Grammy, and we were hoping he'd hear the news of a lifetime at the upcoming awards ceremony. Instead, just over three weeks after giving birth, we found ourselves standing over Macario's fragile, sleeping body in the ICU, wondering if he'd ever walk, speak, or look us in the eye. The bandages framing his tiny skull masked the severity of what he'd just undergone—38 percent of his brain had been removed. What happened in the weeks between these life-changing events was nothing short of every parent's nightmare.

It was Gramps who first saw the signs. In just the first two hours of Macario's arrival home, Gramps and Macario were resting on our couch when Gramps turned to glance at our son. Expecting a sleepy face, what he saw instead will forever be seared in his memory: Macario's eyes were wide open, as if he were staring right through him. Then, he started to foam at the mouth. His body began to seize uncontrollably. Words can't describe the experience of a parent watching their newborn child suffer like this. We rushed him to the emergency room, where the doctors quickly determined he'd had a stroke and was suffering from repeated seizures. As doctors continued to monitor him closely in the hospital, Macario began having around two hundred seizures a day. Macario's doctors said he may have cortical dysplasia, a condition common in epileptic patients. But to us, the *why* didn't matter—we were only focused on the *how*. How could we get our baby to stop seizing? How could we see him through this in a way that could secure him a future free from pain? Was it even going to be possible? Every time I considered Macario's life ahead, a sense of dread would take over my nervous system. Would he have a life at all? *Can our child survive this? Can we?*

If only I knew then what I know now—that Macario would not only recover from his seizures, but that five years later, he'd be a thriving kindergartener, able to speak, run, play at recess, and cuddle with his eternally grateful parents—perhaps I could've saved myself and my family a lot of heartache and grief. But if I'd told my prior self the solution to Macario's critical issues lay in the molecules of a cannabis plant, I would never have believed it.

Like many in my field, I'd spent much of my career not giving cannabis the time of day. It simply wasn't on my radar. The plant may be moving into the mainstream of popular culture at an ever-increasing rate, but the taboo of "weed culture" as "stoner culture" remains strong for many of us. Without thinking too much about the claims of their medicinal value, I simply shrugged hemp and marijuana off the way most do—whether as a vice or as mind-altering entertainment, these drugs didn't have value in my life.

As it turns out, a mother's grief, a gut feeling, and an open mind about learned assumptions can be a particularly potent blend of factors. And in my case, they led me to the most important discovery of my life: a pure CBD oil that not only had the power to heal my son, but to also heal others with drastically different conditions.

> A mother's grief, a gut feeling, and an open mind about learned assumptions can be a particularly potent blend of factors.

In desperation, I created the oil seven months after Macario's birth. Now, my life has a single, monumental mission: give people the tools they need to change their minds about the medicinal value of cannabis and on bridging the gap between the alternative medicine, current medicine, and science. The story of how I found this mission begins with my son's tragedy. But it ends with a victory so big that it could change the world.

MACARIO'S STORY

When I became pregnant with my first child in 2008, I made a simple observation: my gut told me full-time motherhood would not fulfill me, and my brain told me I had a knack for science—and a bachelor's degree in biology and chemistry. After several years of balancing the responsibilities of being a mother of one, then two, with a grueling schedule as a pursuant medical student, then as a PhD candidate, it seemed like a reasonable enough time to make a hypothesis: upon the completion of my doctorate degree, I'd find my way in the scientific community as a cellular biologist, continue to publish my research, and set an example of hard work and determination for my children.

Time seemed to prove my hypothesis. After a divorce from the father of my two eldest children, I'd found an absolutely supportive partner in Gramps Morgan. In addition to being a renowned reggae musician, he was the father of nine incredible kids. Gramps understood the hard work that I was doing because he was doing it himself—on the stage, at the recording studio, and in his own home. Gramps and I had been friends for a long time before we joined families—our strong bond made it feel like anything was possible for us and our eleven kids, and now fourteen children. His support buoyed me through my PhD program and made me feel like my dreams were within reach.

Meanwhile, the mentors I found and the opportunities I was given in my PhD program at Vanderbilt University, first in the neuroscience department, and subsequently in the cardiology and cardio oncology departments, gave me hope that this world was where I belonged. I was part of a grant to study genetic factors that mimicked chemotherapies and their direct effect on heart disease, and over the course of seven years, I presented on my findings. When I had made the switch years earlier from pursuing an MD to pursuing my PhD, I did so with a single focus in mind: I didn't want to simply make diagnoses—I wanted to understand the origins and roots of a problem. Working in developmental biology gave me the opportunity to distill those origins down to a single cell.

If you consider all the steps and ingredients that go into making soup, you could say my work as a cellular biologist—and the work of developmental biologists more generally—was akin to studying just the salt: what it is, what it does, and how every interaction either makes the salt more potent or makes it go away. Then, over time, you move to the next ingredient: you look at the carrot, how it's sliced, what defines it, how it interacts with everything else in the soup. This metaphor came to define my professional life.

For the duration of my PhD program, the fruits of my studies were confined to the size of a petri dish. After seven years, I decided it was time to widen the lens. I had a firm grasp of the cellular origins of specific diseases—I'd studied nearly every tissue-specific cell as well as abnormal cells under the microscope. Now, I wanted to begin to understand how that developmental knowledge and understanding could be translated into specific health outcomes. Translational biology and research is known as the "bench to bedside"[4] bridge—it focuses on using what we know about cell structures to create new medicines and treatment plans for patients. I began the process of obtaining my clinical trial certification around the time Gramps and I became pregnant with our first child together. The certification would help me take what I learned while obtaining my PhD and begin to relate it to the lives of real people. I was always focused on the bigger picture of using my knowledge in a dynamic way to really help the world. By the end of my certification, I'd have the beginning knowledge to be able to engineer clinical trials from the design stage to completion.

Successfully completing my trial certification felt very much like another "experiment" that continued to prove out the hypothesis

---

4   Erin M. Goldblatt, "From bench to bedside: The growing use of translational research in cancer medicine," *American Journal of Translational Research*, 2010; 2(1): 1-18, https://www.ncbi.nlm.nih.gov/pmc/articles/PMC2826819/.

I'd made for my life. That this milestone coincided with Gramps's Grammy nomination and our first pregnancy seemed perfectly serendipitous. We'd already chosen to name our child after the Filipino word for "blessing," and Macario was already living up to his name in the womb. We'd continue to be blessed by Macario's presence in our lives—but in ways I could've never imagined. Just days after the completion of my certification and days before Gramps's Grammy win, Macario's tragedy would prove my hypothesis for my future wrong—and would change our lives for good.

Before the tragedy, there was routine. Every individual is born with innate talents, and I've been blessed with a sense of balance. It had served me well the last few years as I juggled parenting with my PhD program. I'd go to the lab each day, come home, feel tired, set about making dinner, then start all over again. Gramps and I built a steady life.

From January 16 onward, that comfortable routine sailed out the window, replaced by a thick fog of grief and confusion, fear, and panic. It felt unmanageable—and if it weren't for Gramps by my side, maybe it would've been. During those long days at the hospital, we leaned toward each other like never before. When life sends you these huge obstacles, you can attach yourself to your faith. You can pray like you've never prayed in your life—and we did. But having each other to hold, both emotionally and physically, felt like a gift unlike any I'd ever received. There were times I'd collapse into him in tears, comforted only in knowing he was going through the exact same grief as mine.

As a biologist at Vanderbilt, my professional life was adjacent to Macario's suffering. If I had the capacity to research possible solutions for his condition, I would've done so—that kind of thing comes second nature to me. It just wasn't in the cards. In day-to-day life, emotions can often be compartmentalized in order to focus on what's in front of you. What was in front of me now was a child whose condition seemed to be rapidly deteriorating. I was far away from my day-to-day life now. I had to acknowledge my own limitations and place my trust in the medical professionals by our family's side. We watched helplessly as his doctors administered various regimens of prescription medication in an effort to get his seizures under control, and we clung to the moments where they seemed to be working. I remember feeling hopeful one morning when a particular combination of pills had reduced Macario's seizures from the prior night to just two. The very next night, he had fifty. Every new round of medication or new suggestion for changing his diet felt like one step forward, two steps back—there was a complex mixture of answers and emotions and no concrete answer in sight.

A NEUROSURGEON'S OPINION

Three weeks had passed with no clear developments in Macario's condition. We wanted to do right by our child—and yet when we first heard the word "surgery" in our child's hospital room, I ignored the possibility. The neurologists working with Macario were very good, but they'd reached the limits of what they could offer my son. When one of our doctors told me she'd asked the head neurosurgeon to come speak with us, I felt stunned. *We can't do that.* Macario was not even a month old. When I imagined his tiny body on the operating table, the fog overtook me—and it was about to get thicker.

Despite my struggle to accept brain surgery as a possibility, we received a consult from a highly recommended pediatric neurosurgeon at Vanderbilt. His suggestion was as straightforward as it was overwhelming: he had studied Macario's EEG readings and determined that the only way to give our son a chance at a life without seizures was to perform a hemispherectomy—the removal of the entire left hemisphere of his brain—and to do it as quickly as possible. Macario's increasing number of seizures was not a random occurrence: the portions of his brain suffering from these episodes were in effect "training" other areas of his brain to seize as well. This process has been described as the "kindling phenomenon"—a fitting analogy, as the seizures spread like fire throughout the brain until more and more of it appeared to be under siege.[5] There was a sense of urgency rooted in the idea that, if we did not act now, even a hemispherectomy may not be enough to save the remaining healthy neural circuits of Macario's brain.

While my body remained in front of the neurosurgeon as he described the biological basis for his opinion, my mind had entered into another universe as soon as he uttered the word "hemispherectomy." After four weeks of unknowing, this answer provided a path forward yet did not address any questions of what Macario's future might look like. With a growing brain like his, nobody could predict how he would recover or what complications may arise. I'm not sure they wanted to predict any conclusions.

Our brains are incredible instruments. Neuroplasticity, or our brain's ability to reorganize itself and change its structure and function to adapt and survive, is a relatively new field of study—but research continually reaffirms that early childhood is a crucial time for these adaptations to occur.[6] A baby's brain is like a sponge, and its extraor-

---

5   Edward Bertram et al., "The Relevance of Kindling for Human Epilepsy,"
     Epilepsia, 48(Suppl. 2):65–74, 2007, https://onlinelibrary.wiley.com/doi/
     pdf/10.1111/j.1528-1167.2007.01068.x.

6   Patrice Voss et al., "Dynamic Brains and the Changing Rules of Neuroplasticity:
     Implications for Learning and Recovery," *Frontiers in Psychology*, 2017; 8: 1657,
     https://www.ncbi.nlm.nih.gov/pmc/articles/PMC5649212/.

dinary plasticity could work in Macario's favor. And yet, there was no way of knowing how, or if, Macario's brain, once halved, would attempt to reorder itself. Nobody could answer which functions would be lost and which would remain. Nobody could answer whether he'd even survive the surgery.

We've reached a unique point in this era of science and medicine: because our advanced scientific tools have never been more technologically precise, we've come to expect a degree of uniformity or clarity in understanding our own bodies. When we describe our symptoms at the doctor's office, we want to know what they mean and

> There was no way of knowing how, or if, Macario's brain, once halved, would attempt to reorder itself. Nobody could answer which functions would be lost and which would remain.

what we can do about it. It's an understandable ask—but it neglects to factor in a fundamental element of our humanity we are just beginning to understand.

The fact that I recognized the uncertainty inherent to our human condition didn't make Macario's immediate fate any easier to grasp. Every child is different, and every outcome is different. The team at Vanderbilt was realistic and honest in setting these expectations with us. But what was most true did not need to be spoken aloud: once the surgery team removed an entire hemisphere of his brain, Macario would face significant developmental challenges. Not long after he delivered his recommendation, the neurosurgeon left for a neuroscience conference, and we were left to pray that there would be a positive change, a miracle, in Macario before the doctor came back prepared to operate. The prior weeks had been devastating because of the lack of clarity. With Macario's body and brain effectively shut down, our days took on a new dread of knowing what was to come: questions like "What can we do?" were replaced with questions like "Can we really do *this?*"

There was much to be concerned about in thinking of a procedure like this, but my mind kept coming back to the removal of Macario's primary motor cortex, his "motor strip." This portion of the human brain is responsible for our voluntary movements.[7] There were so many what-ifs about removing the entire left hemisphere of his brain. He may not be able to use his right eye. He may not be able to process emotion. The team at Vanderbilt reminded us that nothing was certain. But I knew that, without his motor strip, there was a greater chance he would not develop any motor skills at all.

The neurosurgeon returned from his conference with interesting news that answered my concern: he suggested removing a smaller chunk of Macario's brain, leaving the motor strip intact. The surgery had never been done before, but with his wealth of experience and expertise, there was simply no better person to do it than the presenting neurosurgeon. Gramps and I looked at him as an angel in whom we were instilling so much trust and hope. The risk, however, was that by not removing the entire half, the seizures may persist—and if that occurred, a second brain surgery would likely be required. Gramps and I considered our options: did leaving the door open for Macario to walk and move someday outweigh the potential risk of him having to undergo a second surgery? Even with his motor strip, there was no guarantee Macario would have enough synaptic connectivity to guide this part of the brain to function effectively. But without it, there'd be less of a chance.

---

7   D. Purves et al., "The Primary Motor Cortex: Upper Motor Neurons That Initiate Complex Voluntary Movements," *Neuroscience*, 2nd edition, Sinauer Associates, 2001, https://www.ncbi.nlm.nih.gov/books/NBK10962/.

We knew we were taking a risk by not removing the entire left half—but the risk was impossible to measure. Our hope and the hope of our doctors was that a young developing brain could compensate for his loss, and he could have some form of quality of life. We were expecting to work with Macario for the rest of his life on whatever developmental challenges arose. Gramps and I had been asking ourselves the same question over and over: how are we going to get through this? The question wasn't meant to have an answer. We'd get through this because we had to. We had no other choice. And removing slightly less of Macario's brain would give him the best possible chance.

A LIFESAVING SURGERY—AND WHAT COMES AFTER

On February 10, my son, twenty-eight days old, underwent nine hours of brain surgery. The doctors gave him three blood transfusions, and upon completion, they inserted a gastrostomy tube through his abdomen so he could digest food directly. He was hooked up to so many different IVs and machines that we could barely manage to put our arms around him. The peaceful look of sleep belied the number of medications pumping through his bloodstream. The surgery was successful in that it kept him alive—and for that outcome alone, we were both immeasurably relieved. Only time would tell if it would be enough to prevent his seizures from reoccurring—and months would pass before we'd get a sense of how his postsurgery brain would adjust to its new challenges.

A few short days after Macario's surgery, Gramps and I received our first two blessings since his birth: Gramps won his first Grammy, and we were finally cleared to take Macario home to begin our new life. His time in the hospital postsurgery proved to be seizure free. Time would tell, but it seemed the worst was likely behind us, and for that we were thankful.

The first time we took our son home, we'd anticipated a time of celebration. The second time we took him home, we felt blessed that he'd made it back with us at all. Macario's team of doctors at Vanderbilt planned to keep him on the same medications they'd administered prior to the surgery for an approximate period of two years, at which point Macario would be slowly weaned, or titrated, off the drugs. These meds were potent—and the whole team feared that the seizures would come back if any adjustments were made.

The day after the surgery, a physical therapist visited Macario and suggested a regimen of physical therapy. I had no idea what the therapy would look like for a baby barely a few months old, but our family was so happy after a successful surgery that we obliged every doctor's order. In the next weeks, I dutifully took him to his appointments and administered prescriptions through his G-tube. I struggled through countless sleepless nights listening for the sound of his breathing and anxiously watched for any sign that his seizures would reappear. Months passed, and they never did. It seemed we'd found a new routine.

As a scientist, I may take a methodical approach in my professional life. But in my personal life, I believe strongly that methodology and intellectual rigor have their limits. When my gut tells me something, I trust it. Soon after we'd settled into a routine with Macario with normal feeding and no detection of seizures, I started feeling bothered by his development—or lack thereof. Everyone who met Macario told me what a good baby he was. I'd respond politely, but in my mind, I knew the characteristics they were praising—his calm, quiet, and tear-free demeanor—were just symptoms of his numerous medications, not necessarily his natural personality. By five months, he still acted like a newborn. One day, I looked at Macario and just felt he was capable of more. My gut told me to stop interpreting my son's inability to meet developmental milestones as a side effect of his condition and to start pushing back on the assumption that he may never reach important milestones at all.

When Macario was reeling from his seizures, my own brain was in survival mode. Now that we'd established normalcy, I began wondering how I might use my professional training to serve my son. I've always believed in the impossible and was used to challenging people's ideas of what they claimed couldn't be done. What was possible for Macario's life? It became my mission to find out.

MEANT FOR SOMETHING MORE: WHY I CHOSE CANNABIS FOR MY SON

My gut's intuition that I could do something to help Macario began to feel like an itch I had to scratch—so I began to read anything and everything I could get my hands on that seemed related to his condition. Modern medicine places a laserlike focus on the problem areas of the body and administers prescriptions to target those areas directly. As I reviewed all of the available seizure medications, they all seemed to target one of a few specific pathways in the brain. The drugs acted like a synaptic Band-Aid, tamping down on functionality rather than reviving it. They may be preventing the seizures, but they also weren't allowing for any new growth or development.

Macario's seizures seemed to be under control. Acknowledging the limitations of other seizure meds, and the limitations of targeted medicine more generally, I started to wonder if the ultimate goal should be to wean him off the Band-Aid drugs to give his developmental processes a chance to do their job—and perhaps even find something that would give those synapses a proactive push to advance and grow. I wasn't looking for something that would heal Macario's brain—rather, I was looking for a more holistic solution that would let the body decide what it needed to do to recover—like activate the motor strip we'd preserved or increase cellular communication between his bodily systems. I believed in the power of Macario's internal healing processes, and that belief drove my research toward unexpected places.

> I started to wonder if the ultimate goal should be to wean him off the Band-Aid drugs to give his developmental processes a chance to do their job.

With the mapping of the human genome only recently completed, what's become apparent is as much as our bodies are similar, every individual's genetic makeup is singularly unique. But our genes are only part of the picture. Research is shedding light on the ways in which systems within our bodies are not discrete or contained, but rather continually impact both one another and our mental processes in unpredictable ways.[8] Individuals and cultures have understood this interconnectedness for millennia, but many are just now taking advantage of it outside the doctor's office, focusing on their gut microbiome to manage their multiple sclerosis[9] or using reflexology to cure tension headaches. And just as the systems within our bodies are interconnected, so, too, are the systems at play outside our bodies.

---

8   Sara Reardon, "Gut-brain link grabs neuroscientists," *Nature News*, last updated November 12, 2014, https://www.nature.com/articles/515175a.

9   Sushrut Jangi et al., "Alterations of the human gut biome in multiple sclerosis," *Nature Communications*, last updated June 28, 2016, https://www.nature.com/articles/ncomms12015.

Even if our bodies could be managed with precision, our environments—both physical and social—add a degree of variability that pushes the possibility of predictability even further out of reach. We can build general understanding of possible answers like prescriptions or surgeries, but there are too many unique factors at play to ever be able to fully predict with certainty what will happen. Fifty years from now, this may be different. But for now, we have to accept the truth that's in front of us: a whole lot more goes into our health and wellness than what we currently give our bodies credit for—and there's often not just one easy solution for everyone.

In the beginning stages of my search, cannabis floated around in the back of my mind as a radical idea. I'd read claims that cannabidiol, or CBD—one of hundreds of chemical compounds known as phytocannabinoids found in the cannabis plant—had therapeutic benefits for numerous conditions, including epilepsy. I'd never been particularly interested in this developing field, as my focus was elsewhere, and research on the compound proved to be far from robust. Cannabis as a science never came across my desk. After long nights of reading, however, I couldn't ignore the potential promise of CBD. At the same time, I also couldn't give my son a product unless I knew exactly what was in it. One night, something clicked. I had just received my clinical trial certification—what better time to put it to use than to experimentally analyze some of the CBD products on the market?

CBD is a nonpsychotropic molecule found in abundance in hemp plants, whereas marijuana plants consist primarily of tetrahydrocannabinoidol molecules, or THC, the psychotropic chemicals that produce the high people generally think of when they hear the word *cannabis*. Based on my research, I understood that an isolated form of CBD had a unique ability to naturally interact with the receptors of an individual's endocannabinoid system to bring about homeostasis and internal repair within the body. (We will take a closer look at this system in chapter 3.)

I hypothesized that using CBD to trigger Macario's endocannabinoid system into action would encourage his brain and nervous system to repair on its own and give him a chance to develop by accentuating the processes that would otherwise naturally occur, like the active firing of synapses in the brain to form new and important connections.

Macario's surgery likely threw off the natural homeostasis in his brain and body. I hoped that with the aid of CBD, the body would recognize what needed healing and help trigger his remaining hemisphere's neuroplasticity to compensate for the partial hemisphere that had been removed. By administering CBD straight through Macario's feeding tube, his body would be able to digest the substance more directly than if I fed it to him orally. I needed to find an absolutely pure form of CBD with no residual THC or other cannabinoid molecules; no terpenes, a chemical compound that can give cannabis its distinguishable scent and can alter the way your body processes phytocannabinoids;[10] and no fragrances. It's not that I didn't believe in the other components of the plant, I simply wanted to have a strong starting point that was consistent and pure, so that I could afterward determine what there was to try next—like any other experiment. I needed to find a product that was potentially potent enough to replace Macario's many medications, with a base that could efficiently cross the blood–brain barrier—a requirement for the molecules to effectively reach the endocannabinoid system. A pure, potent CBD oil was what I was after—it seemed like a very simple and logical starting point. And so I began my search.

---

10   Ethan Russo, "Taming THC: Potential cannabis synergy and phytocannabinoid-terpenoid entourage effects," *British Journal of Pharmacology*, 2011 Aug; 163(7): 1344-1364, https://www.ncbi.nlm.nih.gov/pmc/articles/PMC3165946/.

With a clear goal in mind, I used a rented lab and got to work testing several CBD oils just as I'd been trained. I ordered them in packs of three so I could perform a general composition test, in which I'd track their specific dilutions before, during, and after the process. I was looking at three key factors: variability, consistency, and dispersion. Each of these factors was important in determining the product's composition profile, because if I didn't know what exactly was in each CBD bottle, I would not be able to determine proper dosage, nor would I understand what, exactly, was working or not working for Macario and his recovery. What I found during those tests wasn't promising. The minute I put some of the oils into a beaker, I could tell they hadn't been solubilized correctly. They weren't mixed—some even displayed a clumpy texture. I could see with my naked eye they weren't pure and weren't going to be effective.

The entire field of legal cannabis use is so new in our country's history—CBD extracted from hemp plants was only made legal in the United States in 2018, while other forms of cannabis remain illegal in most states and at the federal level. Additionally, the vast majority of products on the market are geared toward recreational rather than medicinal usage, and the regulatory laws on the books reflect that. As just one example, U.S. federal law requires that under 0.3 percent THC is in the final product of CBD oil. But this simply means that while CBD is high and THC is low, the oil may contain a myriad of other cannabinoids with impacts that, although they may be beneficial, haven't been defined and aren't easy to discern. What that translated to in the lab were dozens of minimally regulated products where chemical uniformity varied from bottle to bottle.

It's not the industry's fault: with so little legal oversight and comparatively minimal focus on medicinal use, there hasn't been a reason to bring a prescription-like uniformity to this market. It wasn't the results of the testing or the products themselves that frustrated me—rather, I was frustrated because all the reading I'd done suggested that cannabis would prove to be an effective aid in Macario's development, but a truly transparent CBD just didn't seem to be a product I could buy. I could not risk administering anything less than that to my son, so I decided to stop testing and start creating. If I couldn't buy the CBD I believed could work, I'd have to make it myself. And I did.

> With so little legal oversight and comparatively minimal focus on medicinal use, there hasn't been a reason to bring a prescription-like uniformity to this market.

CREATING MASAYA

Once I realized I couldn't find what I was looking for on the market, I began work creating my own pure CBD formulation. I'd never done anything like this before. My goal with my clinical trial certification was to test new medicines, not create my own. However, based on my understanding of molecular reactivity and chemical composition, it seemed the process of creating a pure CBD formula should be relatively straightforward: I was not trying to throw a hundred ingredients together, I was merely trying to extract one single ingredient and develop a consistent product from that extraction. Nonetheless, I proceeded cautiously. It took me one month of work before I had a product I could test—but once I and others tested it, it passed with flying colors. My CBD oil had zero additional compounds: no terpenes, no THC, no other cannabinoids, nothing. More importantly, I had diluted the CBD in a base that would allow the formulation to have a consistent dispersion rate, bypass the first metabolic pathway, avoiding drug interactions, and cross the blood–brain barrier. I felt so confident in its potency that I took Macario off his other medication cold turkey, replacing them with CBD directly administered through his feeding tube, just as I'd planned.

Within forty-eight hours, Macario's right eye, barely in view due to his missing left occipital lobe, rolled into place. That proved to be just the beginning. He began moving, crawling, and using his right hand, with no abnormalities and thus far exceeding the expectations of his doctors and therapists. Months later, he was walking. Since then, he's checked off every developmental milestone appropriate to his age. He hasn't taken his antiseizure medications since I took him off in 2016.

Three years later, my son is in preschool, and the product that saved his life has saved many others since. Don't get me wrong: the same factors that cause variability in treatment in traditional medicine are still at play with the administration of the CBD oil I developed. I don't think for a second that it was the CBD oil alone that provided such an amazing recovery for Macario. His environment plays a big role: he's growing up with two parents and twelve siblings who love him, along with many teachers, therapists, and close family friends who help to stimulate his successfully developing young body. He has a mother who didn't let doubt stop her from discontinuing the multiple medications that were constantly bombarding his brain. However, I also don't think for a second that CBD didn't play a huge role by encouraging his own bodily resources to spring into action and help his brain recover and rebuild.

The Filipino word for happiness is *masaya*. Happiness is not found in just one place in the mind or body. It emanates from your very being. It's not a cure-all—but it is a potent emotion that helps your whole body and mind recover from hardships, flourish, and truly thrive. I named my CBD oil after this Filipino word. Masaya heals hurting souls by encouraging their body's own healing powers to get to work, rather than acting like a Band-Aid covering their wounds. Masaya acknowledges that our rational minds don't always know, and can't always predict, what will make us better—but we can trust that our *bodies* will know. That's a powerful, revolutionary truth—and I think it's the future of medicine.

* * *

Five years later, my son is in kindergarten. And for the last five years, I've been sharing my story and promoting education to medical professionals and families around the world. This book is not meant to be a calling card for Masaya, however. Rather, it speaks directly to my life's calling: changing people's perceptions and beliefs not only about the power of cannabis, but also about the power of our own bodies, minds, and environments to change our health outcomes.

The medical and scientific fields have come a long way, but we have far to go. I never thought I'd be on this journey, but as I look back, I see how every single decision, every single turn, has led me to this point. Macario, my blessing, turned my world upside down. Now that it's right-side up again, I've never seen my mission more clearly.

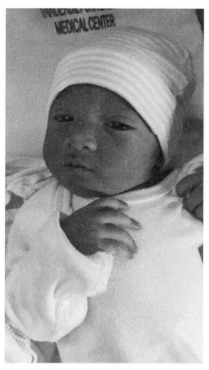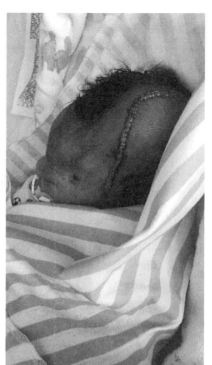
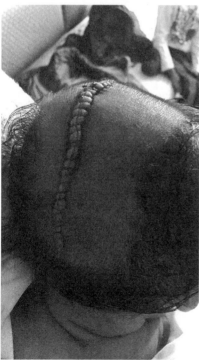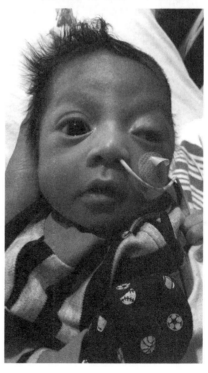

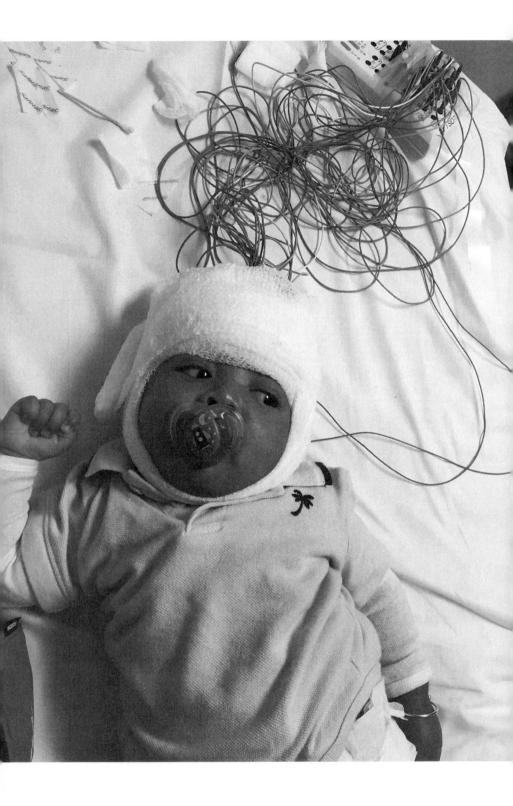

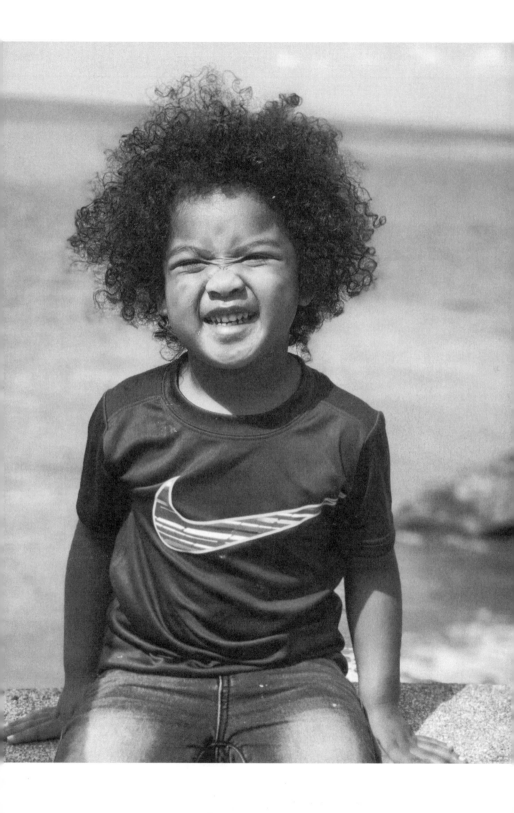

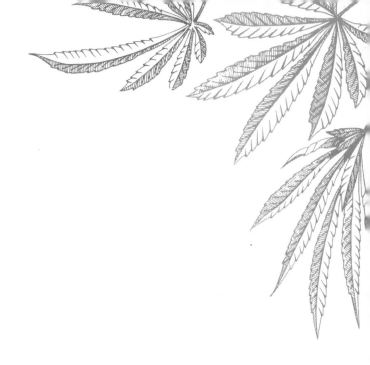

PART ONE

THE CASE FOR CANNABIS

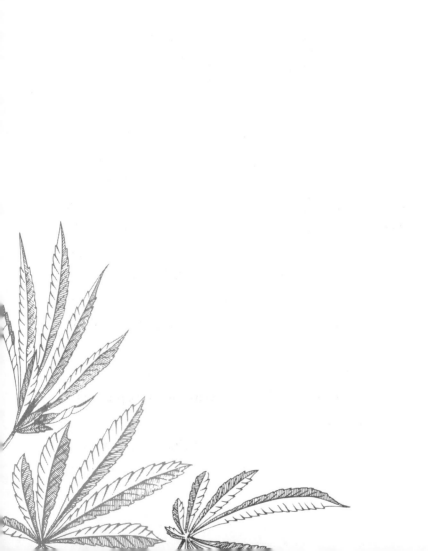

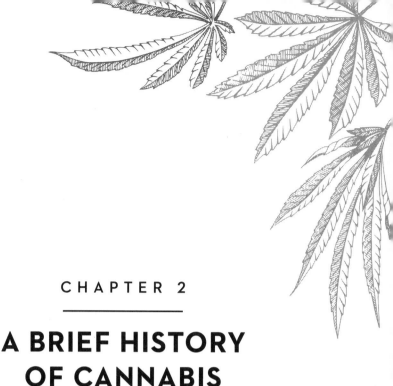

CHAPTER 2

A BRIEF HISTORY
OF CANNABIS

W hen I began my readings on the history and biological benefits of cannabis, I wasn't quite sure
where to start. In my ordinary field of research,
I was used to having a number of studies and
analyses at my fingertips, available with a quick click of the mouse. I
quickly came to find that in the cannabis industry, there simply is no
solid information to pull from—especially on plant medicinal biology.
I had to piece together what I could find and connect the dots as best
as I could. You see, most information we have now of cannabis is
assessed from the outside in, not the inside out—and that presents a
major problem. Let me explain why.

The way things work in my world, medicinal treatments are
assessed from the inside out: first and foremost, researchers would

work toward a solid understanding of the biochemical makeup of a certain substance, breaking it down molecule by molecule and assessing how the molecular structures would interact with human cells to create a chain reaction that would ultimately benefit the health of the patient. There were the molecules in the medicine, and there were the cells of the body, and our research was geared toward understanding how both interacted with one another. Now, nothing in science is ever 100 percent—I often experienced a chain reaction that fixed one problem but created several more in return. But there's a reason certain chemical compounds are sold as prescription medication: they are prescribed to target very specific mechanisms in the body. Results may vary, but they are overwhelmingly effective.

In my research on cannabis, it seemed the plant was being assessed from the outside in: thousands and thousands of articles and internet forums praised the value of cannabis in healing a range of maladies, from seizures to chronic pain to rheumatoid arthritis, and yet I could not find any rigorous research pointing to the biological processes behind these benefits. My frustration was twofold: First, I could find only hints and unfinished research about how cannabis impacted various systems within the body in order to heal. There was no coherent body of work that could take me through the plant biology and the body's biology step by step—there were only fragments. Second, there was a frustrating lack of understanding of basic terminology about the plant. There was hemp and cannabis and marijuana, THC and CBD, indica and sativa, terpenes and cannabinoids, but no single body of work could walk me through what these terms meant, how they related to each other, and most crucially, how they related to the body itself. With the focus so strictly on these buzzwords, they also couldn't tell me what important terms may be missing from my search.

If the medical research I was most familiar with in my work as a biologist could be likened to a peer-reviewed journal article, the insights I found on medical cannabis were like an opinion piece in a local newspaper. I was not used to using first-person anecdotes as a starting point for my work, yet here I was. This descriptive, anecdotal approach to cannabis was directly related to the CBD oils I'd ordered to study in the lab. Biologists know exactly what's in the compounds they study. When I looked at those CBD products under the microscope, it felt like the entire medical marijuana industry was just throwing their substances up against a brick wall and seeing what stuck. And the doctors or physicians in the industry, as positive minded as they were about using cannabis as a medicine and as much progress as they had seen, their claims, the information they were educating on, and the research they knew were all anecdotal as well. Point-blank: proof of effectiveness, quality, and efficiency are completed in the world of science—then played out in a doctor's office. Physician data is after the fact. As a scientist, the information that I was looking for did not exist.

It took me hours and hours of reading before I realized that what Macario needed was not on the market and felt I had enough understanding of what I needed to do in the lab to save him. In the back of my mind, I kept wondering: how did we get here? To some extent I already knew: the cannabis plant is one of the most vilified and misunderstood in the world. After seeing how this plant saved my son, I felt a strong need to lend my voice to setting the record straight, once and for all.

> After seeing how this plant saved my son, I felt a strong need to lend my voice to setting the record straight, once and for all.

DEMYSTIFYING THE "GATEWAY DRUG"

There's an oft-repeated quote that's been passed around so many times it's practically become a platitude: "We fear what we don't understand." While this may be true in certain circumstances, the reality can be a little bit more complicated. I want you to close your eyes for a moment and picture yourself walking down an aisle of over-the-counter medications at your favorite drugstore. You may pass the aspirin, the Benadryl, the ibuprofen, the cough syrup, the Pepto-Bismol. Now, picture handing over a sheet of paper with a prescription scribbled on it to your pharmacist and waiting patiently as the folks behind the counter wrap up that little orange bottle in a paper bag before handing it over to you. As you visualize this scenario, watch what's happening in your body. Do you become tense or fearful? Are you wary or afraid? If you're like me, this scenario is so common that it produces no interior feelings of uncertainty, no second thoughts—just normalcy.

Now, let me ask you another question: do you understand the biological mechanisms behind each of the drugs you pass in the store or the prescriptions you're given at the pharmacy counter? I'm a biologist—this is what I do, it's my world—and even I can't tell you every single one of those mechanisms. We don't understand how these drugs work, but we've been told they do—and we believe that. And as a scientist, I know there are very strict processes that define a product as a medicine long before it even gets behind or over the counter of a pharmacy. There are many instances in this world where we don't understand things, and we rely on outside expertise to fill in the blanks.

Sometimes, however, that outside expertise can steer us wrong.

Now, let's picture another scenario. What appears in your mind's eye when you read the word "cannabis"? Here're some answers that wouldn't surprise me: the image of the sharp jagged leaves of the marijuana plant plastered on an ostentatious banner hanging in a pot dispensary. A joint, wrapped in natural brown paper. A hippie blazing on the beach or on the street, exhaling that distinguishable aroma as you pass. Perhaps you picture a friend staring at you with red eyes, with the look that they're not quite present. Perhaps you imagine, with fear, how getting caught with marijuana can lead to years of jail time. So many of these associations come to us through cultural osmosis—movies like *Pineapple Express* perpetuate the stereotypes. And so much of the baseline feelings of fear have been instilled in us since we were in grade school, learning about the evils of inhaling from our teachers and vowing to ourselves to never, ever get anywhere near the leaf or its by-products—after all, it's the gateway drug.

The lack of understanding around marijuana is not random: in the twentieth century, a number of laws were passed that not only prohibited the plant both recreationally and medicinally, but also limited access to the plant in research labs across the country. This plays out even today: despite the sudden influx of cannabidiol products on the market, CBD is still categorized as a Schedule I controlled substance under the Controlled Substances Act of 1970, meaning it has no accepted medical use, a lack of safety for use under supervision, and a "high potential for abuse."[11]

Our brains are fascinating instruments—and for better or worse, they often take the path of least resistance when it comes to knowledge and ideas. It's much easier not to push back against the stereotypes of weed, or any stereotype pop culture offers us. And yet, this is exactly what life calls us to do. So much of life is uncertain—our futures, our

---

11   Jamie Corroon et al., "Regulatory Status of Cannabidiol in the United States: A Perspective," *Cannabis and Cannabinoid Research*, 2018; 3(1): 190–194, https://www.ncbi.nlm.nih.gov/pmc/articles/PMC6154432/.

bank accounts, our romantic prospects—and it feels safe to let others determine the limits of our own understanding. But maturity requires us to live in the shades of gray. Much of our adult lives are a process of unlearning. And the more each of us does the hard work of pushing back, the better our culture is for it.

Cannabis is the most commonly cultivated illicit drug worldwide, and according to the World Health Organization, over 2.5 percent of the entire global population consumes it annually.[12] I found out about this statistic once I had already seen Macario flourish—and it shocked me. The stat also bothered me because I now know there is a serious lack of research, even though there are billions of people that can benefit from it. Billions of dollars are being dumped into the industry, but not into proper science.

> What if we could think of the marijuana plant like we think of the fungus that gave us penicillin—as just a regular old plant with some marvelous healing benefits?

What if we could think of the marijuana plant like we think of the fungus that gave us penicillin—as just a regular old plant with some marvelous healing benefits? What if we could demystify the image of this pointy-leaved plant so that when we see it displayed on a sign or a bottle, it was more akin to seeing the image of a daisy on a T-shirt design?

"We fear what we don't understand" may be a somewhat misleading aphorism, but I can tell you one that's not: those who can't remember the past are condemned to repeat it. The problem with not pushing back against what you've been taught or

---

12   Mary Barna Bridgeman et al., "Medicinal Cannabis: History, Pharmacology and Implications for the Acute Care Setting," *Pharmacy and Therapeutics*, 2017 Mar; 42(3), 180–188, https://www.ncbi.nlm.nih.gov/pmc/articles/PMC5312634/.

learned through cultural osmosis is that so often those understandings are just the tip of the iceberg. When you see a marijuana leaf and think, "that's what gets you high," your mind swiftly negates thousands of years of history—and a much broader and more interesting historical usage. Revealing the origins of this misunderstood plant's usage is the first step in debunking its strange power over our culture. And the origins begin over five thousand years ago.

WHAT DID OUR ANCESTORS KNOW?

Growing up in Saskatchewan, learning native Indian medicinal practices and spirituality in a Filipino household where natural preventative supplementation and natural remedies always were tried before going to a concrete building to get a prescription from a man with a white coat, I have always had a special place in my heart for the power of the healing ways of the past. And I always knew that what we know today had to start somewhere. Additionally, different parts of the earth had different beliefs but they, like religion, had such similar end games, and ultimately medicine was simply about how to heal.

My frustrating search for medical studies led me to look into the history of the plant. I, too, wanted to end up with an amazing anecdotal story for my son, but I needed to know so much more about it. The diversity of this plant, on the molecular level, became such a fascinating subject of interest to me because I had never heard of a species that could provide so many things.

According to historical studies, the cannabis plant may be the oldest plant *not* grown specifically for food—but this extremely versatile plant was used for that too. The hemp seed, or the seed of the cannabis sativa plant, was so commonplace in ancient China that it was considered one of the five staple grains, along with rice, barley, millet, and soy beans. China was certainly not the only ancient culture that used the hemp plant not just for food but for its sturdy fiber, which continues to be a valuable resource in making rope and other textiles. But it was in China that the first recorded medicinal use of the plant occurred. The Pen-ts'ao Ching, the earliest book of Chinese medicine, was compiled in 100 CE but dates back to c. 2700 BCE and is attributed to Emperor Shen Neng. Known as the father of Chinese medicine, Shen Neng knew very well this plant had psychotropic qualities. His book states, "Ma fen [cannabis], if taken in excess, will produce hallucinations. If taken over a long term, [it] makes one communicate with spirits and lightens one's body."[13] However, he also knew its medicinal, nonpsychotropic benefits: he prescribed a cannabis tea for the treatment of rheumatism, malaria, gout, and even poor memory.[14]

Chinese medical texts, including the Pen-ts'ao Ching, recorded usage of every part of the cannabis plant, from the leaf to the root to the water used to process the stalk into fiber.[15] Food, fiber, hallucinogenic, and medicine—China was one among many cultures that acknowledged the multiplicity of uses without vilification. It was also one among many that recognized the potent spiritual aspects of the plant. Burned cannabis seeds have been found in shaman graves from the Middle East to North Africa. Cannabis terpenes, the organic compounds that give the plant its aromatic smell, have been used in

---

13   Mia Touw, "The Religious and Medicinal Uses of Cannabis in China, India and Tibet," *Journal of Psychoactive Drugs*, Volume 13(1), Jan–March, 1981, https://www.cnspro-ductions.com/pdf/Touw.pdf.

14   Peter A. Clark et al., "Medical marijuana: Medical necessity versus political agenda," *Medical Science Monitor*, 2011; 17(12): RA249–RA261, https://www.ncbi.nlm.nih.gov/pmc/articles/PMC3628147/.

15   E. Joseph Brand et al., "Cannabis in Chinese Medicine: Are Some Traditional Indications Referenced in Ancient Literature Related to Cannabinoids?," *Frontiers in Pharmacology*, 2017; 8: 108, https://www.ncbi.nlm.nih.gov/pmc/articles/PMC5345167/.

spiritual practice in the form of incense or smoke for thousands of years—and continue to be used today in numerous countries, as we'll discuss in chapter 7. But one country in particular was so intricately familiar with this plant that it featured in its most sacred legends. Home to some of the most sophisticated understandings of natural medicine in the world, India's ancient Ayurvedic texts noted cannabis as one of the five sacred herbs.[16] In fact, it is in India where the United States' own history of medical cannabis usage begins.

INDIA'S CANNABIS LEGACY

The *Samudra Manthan,*[17] or the Churning of the Ocean of Milk, is one of the best-known legends in Hindu philosophy. The story describes an epic battle between divinities and demons as they search for the nectar of immortality. The search begins when the devas, or divinities, receive a curse that deprives them of their strength, and the asuras, or demons, win control of the universe. The devas go to Lord Vishnu for help, who tells them to seek out the nectar of immortality that resides at the bottom of the Ocean of Milk. Given their lack of strength, the devas would need assistance—so they recruit the asuras, luring them with the possibility of winning the nectar from the bottom of the sea. Using a mountain as a churning rod and a snake as the rope, the asuras and the devas churned for one thousand years. After some time, a poison called *halahala* emerged from the ocean—Lord Shiva drank the poison to protect

---

16   "Ayurvedic View of Marijuana," Soma Matha Organization, accessed April 2020, http://www.somamatha.org/ayurvedic-view-of-marijuana.html.

17   "The story of samundra manthan: The churning of the celestial ocean of milk," Naresh Agarwal, accessed April 2020, http://slis.simmons.edu/blogs/naresh/2014/03/08/the-story-of-samundra-manthan-the-churning-of-the-celestial-ocean-of-milk/.

the universe. The poison turned his throat the characteristic blue that Shiva is known for throughout India and the world. As the legend has it, to save him from his death, he was offered *bhang*—a cannabis-infused drink made from the leaves of the plant that has been consumed in India since at least 1000 BCE and continues to be consumed regularly throughout the country today. According to another interpretation, when the nectar of immortality finally emerged, a drop hit the surface of the earth and a cannabis plant sprouted on the spot.[18]

Thanks to its association with religion, spirituality, and healing, cannabis as medicine truly came into its own in India.[19] In addition to its place in the legend of the Ocean of Milk, cannabis was also recognized in India's most sacred texts, the *Vedas*, as a "liberator," "joy giver," and "source of happiness." The *Atharva Veda* named it one of the five sacred plants, and it was used in Ayurveda for memory problems, leprosy, and much more. Interestingly, academics in this area suggest that

"medicinal [cannabis] use was not originally distinguished from religious use. The reference in the Atharva Veda *to overcoming enemies and evil forces may, quite possibly, have included physical as well as spiritual ills. Once medicinal use became increasingly delimited from religious use, it remained distinct from secular use and could, therefore, be freely and fully explored unhampered by secrecy or disreputability."*[20]

---

18   Mia Touw, "The Religious and Medicinal Uses of Cannabis in China, India and Tibet," *Journal of Psychoactive Drugs*, Volume 13(1), Jan–March, 1981, https://www.cnsproductions.com/pdf/Touw.pdf.

19   Ibid, https://www.cnsproductions.com/pdf/Touw.pdf.

20   Ibid, https://www.cnsproductions.com/pdf/Touw.pdf.

Equally of interest, Ayurvedic doctors prefer to administer cannabis over opium when treating severe pain, because cannabis does not have as many side effects.[21]

In contemporary India, there's technically a single acre of land where cannabis can grow legally. That acre belongs to the Indian Institute of Integrative Medicine, where scientists grow the plant with increased optimism about its medical benefits. While the law prevents possession of cannabis, and consuming it can lead to six months of jail time, cannabis naturally grows all over the subcontinent, and people regularly consume its fruits, using the seeds in chutneys and the fiber to make fabrics.[22] The Narcotic Drugs and Psychotropic Substances Act of 1985 prevents the production, sale, and consumption of certain parts of the plant, but the cannabis leaves remain the exception—bhang is simply too embedded in the culture. In fact, there are even government-approved bhang shops where people can buy the drink and benefit from its healing properties.[23]

O'SHAUGHNESSY'S INFLUENCE

The Sanskrit word for cannabis is *vijaya*, or victory. The contemporary government was not the first source of power in India that couldn't stomach taking this victorious drink away from the people of India. When the British took power in India in the eighteenth

---

21 Amrit Dhillon, "India's history of cannabis use encourages scientists to explore new ways of using it as a legal painkiller," *South China Morning Post*, December 26, 2018, https://www.scmp.com/lifestyle/health-wellness/article/2179351/indias-history-cannabis-use-encourages-scientists-explore.

22 Ibid, https://www.scmp.com/lifestyle/health-wellness/article/2179351/indias-history-cannabis-use-encourages-scientists-explore.

23 Charukesi Ramadurai, "The intoxicating drug of an Indian god," BBC, last updated March 13, 2017, http://www.bbc.com/travel/story/20170307-the-intoxicating-drug-of-an-indian-god.

century, the ubiquitous use of bhang was shocking to them. In ste-reotypically Western fashion, they commissioned a study to better understand the effects and significance of the drug. The results were simply put: "To forbid or even seriously restrict the use of so holy and gracious an herb as the hemp would cause widespread suffering and annoyance … it would rob people of solace in discomfort, a cure in sickness, of a guardian whose gracious protection saves them from attacks of evil influences."[24]

During this period of rule, an Irish chemist and toxicologist named Dr. William Brooke O'Shaughnessy traveled with the British East India Company to Bengal to learn about Ayurveda. He was a brilliant mind and well respected in his home country, and would eventually become the first chemistry professor at Calcutta Medical College. He took an especially curious interest in the cannabis plant and began experiment-ing to determine the extent of its healing properties. His work showed that cannabis could aid in a wide range of maladies, from cholera to rheumatic diseases to infantile convulsions—like the ones my own son experienced nearly two centuries later.

O'Shaughnessy took his work extremely seriously, and his investigative approach was quite sophisticated: he introduced the botanical description of cannabis, documented its many preparations in India, and gave a historical overview of the plant through time. His resulting report, published in a significant treatise entitled "Extract from a memoir on the Preparations of the Indian Hemp, or Gunjah (Cannabis indica), their effects on the animal system in Health, and their utility in the treatment of Tetanus and other Convulsive Diseases, in two parts in one regional journal," became a watershed

---

24   J. M. Campbell, "Report of the Indian Hemp Drugs Commission, 1894–1895," *India Papers*, volume 3, page 252, https://digital.nls.uk/indiapapers/browse/archive/74552222?&mode=zoom)&_sm_au_=iVVnrnkRJ6HStjGn.

moment in the history of medical cannabis, earning O'Shaughnessy the reputation as "the father of modern medical cannabis."[25]

Dr. O'Shaughnessy brought his research back to England, where it made significant waves in the medical world. His research making it to the shores of the United States in the mid-1800s marked the beginning of that country's twisted history with medical cannabis.

CANNABIS COMES TO THE UNITED STATES

Thanks to O'Shaughnessy's research and interest in cannabis in India, cannabis as medicine appeared for the first time in the *United States Pharmacopeia* in 1850. An important resource even today, the annual *Pharmacopeia* is a compilation of drug information that sets standards of strength, quality, and purity for pharmaceuticals. Under its 1850 listing, cannabis was described as a treatment for everything from menstrual bleeding to rabies, incontinence, gout, and both alcohol and opioid addiction. At this point, the drug had no politics about it: it was simply a useful cure to numerous ails. By 1937, things had changed.

The Marijuana Tax Act of 1937 was the first of several politically complicated pieces of legislation against a plant with proven medical benefits. The act, which heavily taxed hemp products, was the result of numerous outside forces working against cannabis, many of which sound eerily familiar in the contemporary era of the United States: there was fear sparked by Mexican immigrants, who introduced the culture to the recreational use of marijuana, and

---

25 Ethan B. Russo, *History of Cannabis as Medicine: Nineteenth Century Irish Physicians and Correlations of Their Observations to Modern Research*, New York: Springer International Publishing, 2017, https://www.semanticscholar.org/paper/Chapter-2-History-of-Cannabis-as-Medicine-%3A-Century-WilliamBrooke-Shaughnessy/90a d7a72b679b4f80f1d3f59dfdb648c6c8c280d.

subsequent propaganda, like the movie *Reefer Madness* in 1936, that stoked the racialized fears of the public. And there were capitalist forces at play. The DuPont family had just introduced the synthetic fiber nylon to the market and found natural hemp fiber to be its most significant competitor. Randolph Hearst, another wealthy man, worried that hemp fibers would soon replace paper pulp in his newspapers—and he had significant timber holdings that could feel the financial pinch of lost business.[26]

Ancient China, ancient and modern-day India, and many cultures in between have been able to hold the complexities of this multi-dimensional plant without diminishing its usefulness and without introducing mass hysteria or fear. The United States has not done the same, and in bowing to the fear, we've reduced a complex medicine to its basest stereotype.

This is the story most of us already know: as the populace began internalizing the hysteria, the government heightened restrictions and penalties. The *Pharmacopeia* dropped medical cannabis from its text in 1942. The Boggs and the Narcotic Control Acts increased penalties for cannabis possession in 1951 and 1956, respectively. In 1970, the Controlled Substances Act classified cannabis as a Schedule I substance, a recognition reserved for drugs with a high potential of abuse and no accepted medical use. These legislative actions gave oxygen to the cultural stereotypes persisting throughout the twentieth century, emphasizing that the only power of this plant was as a form of mind-altering entertainment or counterculture "enlightenment." Meanwhile, they sucked all of the air out of the room for any further research. Beyond mere criminalization, the

---

26   Laurence French et al., *NAFTA and Neocolonialism: Comparative Criminal, Human and Social Justice*, Lanham, Maryland: University Press of America, Inc., 2004, page 129, https://books.google.com/books?id=4ozF1Yg-c4MC&pg=PA129#v=onepage& q&f=false.

new laws limited scientific research by restricting procurement of the plant even for academic reasons.[27]

In 1996, California legalized medical use of cannabis for severe or chronic illnesses in its Compassionate Use Act. Since then, cannabis has been increasingly decriminalized. But in many instances, we're no longer ingesting the same cannabis—the plant itself has been modified to suit our entertainment needs, rather than our medical needs. In the midnineties, confiscated plants had just 4 percent THC. In 2014, this number had tripled to 12 percent. Now, some products are as high as 37 percent THC. THC has valuable potential as a treatment for nausea and pain—but the increase in THC is not medically necessary. Medical marijuana has been legalized in over half the country, and yet the plants on the market are overwhelmingly produced to serve a different purpose.

To some, "medical marijuana" remains an oxymoron. Even just ten years ago, "weed doctors" would give you a medical card for practically anything—allowing you to visit any dispensary to buy any product. Now, CBD is catching on as the next hottest product on the market, yet the medical cannabis industry remains in a continuing state of relative disarray.

Dr. O'Shaughnessy had the right idea two centuries ago, when he set about understanding this plant from both a cultural and chemical standpoint—and like any good scientist, he did so without any preconceived notions or biases acting as inputs in his research. If our current industry is in a state of disarray, could a turn back to science and biology pave the way for a different future? That's my hope— and that's why, like O'Shaughnessy, I want to give you the scientific backdrop of this incredible plant.

---

27   Mary Barna Bridgeman et al., "Medicinal Cannabis: History, Pharmacology, and Implications for the Acute Care Setting," *Pharmacy and Therapeutics*, March 2017; 42(3): 180–188, https://www.ncbi.nlm.nih.gov/pmc/articles/PMC5312634/.

SHOULD CANNABIS BE CONTROVERSIAL?

In America, scientists who want to conduct research into cannabis must jump through a series of convoluted regulatory steps and review processes involving the National Institute on Drug Abuse (NIDA), the US Food and Drug Administration (FDA), and the US Drug Enforcement Administration (DEA), to name just a few organizations that may be involved. And in most other countries, it's similarly a very extensive and confusing process.

Currently, cannabis for research purposes can only be obtained through NIDA, which sources all of their cannabis from the University of Mississippi. It's an almost laughably archaic system, given the glut of products on the market currently—but in reality, the lack of resources and research is no laughing matter. Much, much more research needs to be done before any scientist could reliably provide a sweeping view of cannabis's range of benefits in the way O'Shaughnessy provided with his more rudimentary scientific tools in the 1830s. Given the tools we have now, O'Shaughnessy's research just scratched the surface of what we might discover about this plant.

While the research catches up to our technological advancements and slowly opening minds and legal framework, what I can begin to provide here is a biologist's viewpoint on the plant: the molecular differences between cannabis species, the chemical composition, and—in the next chapter—how that chemical composition directly impacts our bodies.

THE TAXONOMY DEBATE

Scientific taxonomy offers a useful way to begin to consider the cannabis plant. Biological taxonomy organizes groups of organisms according to shared characteristics, creating smaller and more specific groups until reaching a singular, unique species. Those groups are known as domains: domain, kingdom, phylum, class, order, family, genus, and species. Domain, the broadest, is the most simple: all living species with a nucleus containing genetic information are qualified as eukarya (the other two groups are bacteria and archaea, which display differences in their membranes). Cannabis is a green, flowering organism—so it belongs to the plant kingdom. Phylum, class, and order are similarly large umbrellas for a number of species that share generic qualities. Cannabis's order, Rosales, relates it to roses, strawberries, elms, figs, and nettles.

Its family specifies cannabis even further still. The only two notable genera in this family are cannabis and humulus—the latter, colloquially known as "hops," are what give beer its bitter flavor. *Cannabis* is a genus. As a useful framework, other examples of genera include *rosa* (which provides the umbrella term for over one hundred species, including the California wild rose and the sweetbriar rose), *equus* (of which horses and zebras are both a part), and *panthera* (of which the lion, jaguar, leopard, and tiger are all a part). Species is the most specific classification of any living thing: organisms of the same species can exchange genes and interbreed. The scientific naming system names the genus and the species both: *Panthera tigris* for the tiger; *Panthera leo* for the lion; *Panthera onca* for the jaguar. So, too, does the genus *cannabis* follow this structure: *Cannabis indica, Cannabis sativa*, and *Cannabis ruderalis* are all said to be species of the cannabis plant. However, nothing is straightforward at this stage in our cannabis research—and that extends even into the speciation of the plant.

Under the genus *Cannabis*, there are two familiar species: *Cannabis sativa* and *Cannabis indica*. These terms are meant to define a marijuana or hemp plant for their differences. However, science is getting away from this categorization because these terms cause confusion, and on a molecular level cannabis is far too complex to be pushed into two or sometimes three categories. Nevertheless, hemp and marijuana are both from the *Cannabis* genus and differ by their molecular compositions—those very cannabinoids that either produce a medicinal or a psychoactive effect, or both. From appearance alone, it makes sense these two species have been differentiated from one another. Physically, hemp grows taller and stockier in the fields. Its fibrous, canelike structure was cultivated by civilizations across history, who used it to make clothing, rope, and other important substances. Marijuana appears branchier, or leafier, in the field. However, due to the restrictions on cannabis research, there remain precious few scientific resources that help determine the evolution and speciation of this plant—and whether these differences are significant enough to warrant separation on a species level.

This confusion has a long history, beginning in 1783, when French biologist Jean-Baptiste Lamarck first suggested separating the plants into the indica and sativa categories, based on both their variant morphologies and their variant psychoactive impacts.[28] The issue has been a subject of contentious debate since then. In 2005, contemporary research proposed a similar division based on an allozyme variation within the genus, which is a structural difference at the enzymatic level, not a functional one,[29] but most

---

28   Jacob L. Erkelens et al., "That which we call Indica, by any other name would smell as sweet," *Cannabinoids*, 2014; 9(1): 9–15, https://bedrocan.com/wp-content/uploads/2014-that-which-we-call-indica-by-any-other-name-hazekamp-erkelens.pdf.

29   Jason Sawler et al., "The Genetic Structure of Marijuana and Hemp," *Public Library of Science One*, 2015; 10(8): e0133292, https://www.ncbi.nlm.nih.gov/pmc/articles/PMC4550350/.

other scientists believe that the indica/sativa dichotomy should be abandoned. Again, the majority opinion would consider cannabis as a monotype, with no differences significant enough to warrant speciation outside of the broad umbrella of *Cannabis sativa L.* All forms of cannabis are simply a biochemical mix of the same species.

Making things ever more complicated, *indica* and *sativa* are well known among recreational cannabis users as two different "strains" of cannabis that offer two very different "highs." Any recreational pot shop employee could tell you that their indica strains will lead to a more relaxed high, while sativa produces more of an energetic euphoria. However, these categorizations are not scientifically based—rather, they're descriptive. One Colorado-based dispensary CEO described the classification of weed strains as an art, not a science. As he put it, he can tell the difference between strains by smoking or ingesting the weed and observing if he'd rather be sprawled out on the couch or philosophizing about life. If the former, it's indica. If the latter, it's sativa.[30] It's safe to say scientists of any department would not be particularly pleased about this "artful" classification process. I, however, have no fixed opinion on these categorizations. Medically, it doesn't make sense to utilize that classification, but as in history, if one finds a spiritual balance or awakening from the plant, I believe that should be a freedom they should be responsibly able to take advantage of. There is simply too much confusion within the space of cannabis in general, and the indica/sativa terminology is clearly a categorization for the recreational user. My interest is the science and the gaps that this confusion has created.

---

30 Shannon Palus, "The Indica vs. Sativa Distinction Isn't Real," *Slate*, last updated April 20, 2019, https://slate.com/technology/2019/04/indica-sativa-difference-cannabis-weed-science.html.

THE MOLECULAR BACKGROUND OF CANNABIS

Recreational terminology and interbreeding to produce higher levels of THC has distracted the scientific understanding of the plant and is forcing science to ignore the noise and move backward, or start from the root.

In some ways, the debate in academic circles around the indica/sativa dichotomy, and the way the recreational cannabis world has co-opted these terms for both marketing and "characterizing your high" purposes, encapsulates the widespread confusion that continues to be perpetuated. The blatant contrast between research and marketing also appears at the molecular level of the cannabis plant. Just as recreational users are familiar with indica and sativa, they'll undoubtedly recognize THC and CBD—the two most well-known chemical compounds of the cannabis plant. These chemical compounds are known as cannabinoids, and are so named because of their unique interaction with our body's endocannabinoid system—we'll cover that system in the next chapter.

> **CBD is nonpsychoactive, found in large amounts in hemp, and has far-ranging benefits we are only beginning to fully acknowledge.**

Tetrahydrocannabinol, or THC, is the primary psychoactive compound in the cannabis plant, and is found in large amounts in marijuana. As we'll see in chapter 3, it also interacts with our cannabinoid receptors in ways that can have significant medical benefits. Cannabidiol, or CBD, is nonpsychoactive, found in large amounts in hemp, and has far-ranging benefits we are only beginning to fully acknowledge. Macario is just one example of many who have been healed from this potent cannabinoid.

The recreational cannabis world has jumped on these terms as a key marketing strategy—and yet, the cannabis plant is not just THC or CBD. In fact, there are over one hundred other identified cannabinoids, terpenes, and other compounds found in the glandular trichomes of the cannabis plant flowers. If THC and CBD are powerhouses, it's likely because they are conveniently abundant in cannabis and the only two cannabinoids we've chosen to place our focus on. In our emphasis of these two chemical compounds, what might we be missing from the other hundred compounds extant in the cannabis plant?

The CBD oil I created was a pure distillation of a single cannabinoid. Almost every other product on the market—both those marketed as medical as well as recreational—is not a pure compound. As we will discuss further in chapter 5, there is a popular idea that a whole plant or an extract that is comprised of more of the cannabinoids provide an entourage benefit or synergistic effect. It makes sense—more of the plant working together to provide a catalyst effect to the most potent cannabinoid. I'm not at all against the idea of this ideology becoming a possibility. But the problem is that we have not appropriately defined more than six or seven of these plant molecules/cannabinoids—not alone and certainly not in interaction with other components of the plants and then with the body in order to make such a claim. Terms like the entourage effect try to make the biology of the plant sound simple when, in fact, the biology of both plant and body display a complexity we don't yet have the tools to fully understand.

As a cellular biologist, it's hard for me to understand how the medical industry is comfortably able to prescribe, or in this case, recommend a substance to a patient without knowing its molecular basis and functionality in its entirety. I do feel like cannabis is overall safe, but there are so many unknowns. The problem I fear is that without proper education, these complex, fascinating chemical compounds will be reduced to marketing jargon. When products flood the market with no regulation or clarity around what they contain, people will experience varying results—like what I found in my analysis of CBD oils—and they will quickly lose faith in these substance's power to heal. We'll look more closely at this industry crisis in chapter 4 and beyond.

* * *

Cannabis is one of the oldest known plants to be cultivated by civilizations across the world. From China to India to our own shores in the United States, the unique properties of this plant have been widely acknowledged—and widely feared. We fear what we don't understand—but when cultural misunderstandings remain widespread, there's little opportunity for the truth to be revealed. The stigmatization of cannabis has limited its usefulness in our culture and beyond. Now that I've taken as much of an understanding to its chemical makeup as possible based on what is available in depth, I have a different fear than most: that if we do not stop the perpetuation of the myths surrounding this plant, we may deprive countless individuals of an opportunity to heal their bodies. Macario was my miracle—what other miracles might occur, if only we as a society were brave enough to change our perceptions?

Many of the doctors sending their patients to cannabis dispensaries don't realize that hemp is cannabis, or that hemp and marijuana are on so many levels the same. Most don't realize that not all of the components of this plant are psychoactive, or that impure CBD oils aren't potent enough to bring about the results many of the marketing materials proclaim. When it comes to medical cannabis, we understand far less than we should, especially when this is such a popular and growing industry. Many of the marketing claims reach far beyond the research that's available to us. This is no single entity's fault: it's just the reality of the industry. That doesn't mean we can't do something about it—and we should. The impetus for that change likely lies in understanding more about the system responsible for processing cannabis: the endocannabinoid system.

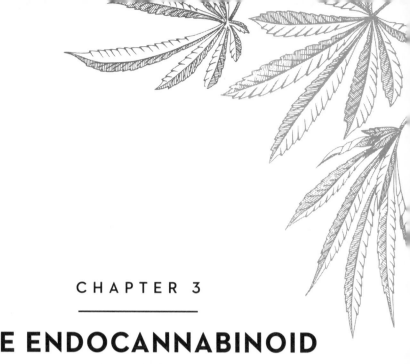

CHAPTER 3

THE ENDOCANNABINOID SYSTEM

When we decided with our team of doctors to remove 38 percent of my newborn son's brain, my world was full of what-ifs. Macario would have no chance to regrow the developing neurons he lost—but what would the remaining neurons in a growing brain become capable of? Would the remaining areas of his brain compensate for the loss? We preserved his brain's motor strip—but this was by no means a guarantee he would exhibit any motor functionality as he grew.

In my work as a scientist, I've studied some of the strictest systems in the body. Both the brain and the heart are developmentally patterned in a very timely manner, and are quite characterized when it comes to cell type composition and cell signaling. This means there is a tightly ordered process that can define the milestones of organ development. Science has allowed this patterning to be quite predictable. Additionally, after the development phase, the functionality of an organ is so well defined, abnormalities have become easier to identify and characterize.

Part of what makes these two organs unique is the cells that render them functional: the brain's neurons and the heart's myocytes don't divide further after development—that is, we don't make new ones. What we're born with is what we've got. And both of these cell types are the most abundant of their organ types. This explains why it is so difficult to come back from neurological or cardiac injury. While nearly every other type of cell in our bodies can rejuvenate themselves, our major brain and heart cells just don't have the capability.

These systems are quite hard-wired—but that doesn't always make them predictable. Macario's surgery was the perfect example of this fact. This certain uncertainty is both the beauty and terror of my field, and our lives: in our sophisticated, high-tech world, where every answer feels within our reach at the click of a mouse, each and every one of us still must grapple with the truth of our human condition. You can set a control for nearly everything, but when it comes to the final outcome, *you cannot guarantee anything.*

Ancient civilizations were more comfortable with the divine mystery of the universe. But since the advent of modern science, that mystery has been rendered unacceptable by many in my profession. I'm guilty of it too—the need to know, the need to understand. The perfect repetition in the outcome of data. And yet, my experience has shaped me in such a way that I also understand the limitations of this viewpoint. Knowledge is power—but sometimes, when we get too comfortable with what we think we know, we miss deep truths lying just beneath our noses. There's something to be said for getting comfortable with a little discomfort in my line of work, and remaining open to the unexplored areas of our lives and bodies, waiting to reveal themselves.

The human body has been the object of fascination to philosophers and scientists since time immemorial. Our rudimentary understanding of many of our body systems are rooted in knowledge acquired and passed on from thousands of years ago: the ancient Greeks attempted an understanding of our nervous system in the fifth century BCE. The Enlightenment era in Europe ushered in many discoveries about our systems that remain unargued even today. But despite our physical bodies being discrete entities, we are still learning so much about how they operate—and what they are capable of. One of the most fascinating discoveries about our bodies—and possibly one of the most consequential—occurred just thirty years ago, when scientists first isolated and cloned a cannabinoid receptor.[31] CB1 proved a decades-old theory of a bodily system unlike any other. It seems the magic of the cannabis plant does not lie in the plant alone—rather, it fits like a puzzle piece into a system that can interpret its compounds and put them to work. The system is named after the compounds themselves, despite being present in human and other animal bodies well before we knew to harvest cannabis medicinally or otherwise: in this chapter, we'll be taking an in-depth look into the endocannabinoid system.

> It seems the magic of the cannabis plant does not lie in the plant alone— rather, it fits like a puzzle piece into a system that can interpret its compounds and put them to work.

---

31   Bradley E. Alger, "Getting High on the Endocannabinoid System," *Cerebrum*, November 1, 2013, https://www.ncbi.nlm.nih.gov/pmc/articles/PMC3997295/.

CHANGE DOESN'T COME EASY— ESPECIALLY IN SCIENCE

In many ways, the functionality of the endocannabinoid system begins to answer so many of the cannabis plant's greatest mysteries. It is within this system that we may begin to measure the unique capabilities of each of the plant's many cannabinoids. It's also within this system that researchers have the opportunity to understand with greater clarity the discrete differences between the most well-known cannabinoids, THC and CBD, and why inhalation or ingestion of these two compounds may lead to different outcomes. And yet, when you look up the endocannabinoid system on Google—just as when you look up sativa, indica, THC, CBD, or any of the numerous buzzwords we covered in the prior chapter—the first results that appear are marketing materials from dispensaries. As smart consumers, we're trained to take such materials with a grain of salt. We assume what they tell us is only half true—and sure enough, if you click through some of those materials, you begin to spot unproven claims, assumptions, or misunderstandings. I understand why this is—but I also realize the significance of the insights that are getting lost in the marketing shuffle, and I wish it wasn't so.

Nearly every major scientific discovery has had to reckon with popularly held beliefs that directly contradict their novel claims. The reason for this is simple: as humans, we structure our lives around collectively held truths, norms, and taboos. When one of those truths suddenly gets dismantled, societies scramble to adjust. The path of least resistance is often to refuse new insights altogether—or render them useless by indifference or ignorance.

The endocannabinoid system is so fascinating and promising that it should be sitting at the forefront of scientific research and funding initiatives. And yet, nearly thirty years after its existence was confirmed, physicians and scientists alike remain unaware of its existence—and I believe this could very well be because of the way cannabis-as-entertainment has stolen the spotlight. This is both concerning and unsurprising. In fact, I consider it the twenty-first century's answer to a centuries-old problem in scientific discovery.

WILLIAM HARVEY AND THE CIRCULATORY SYSTEM: A PARABLE

Of the many body systems to be discovered during the Enlightenment era, the discovery of the true nature of our circulatory system came at a particularly interesting time in history. In the early seventeenth century, its discoverer, William Harvey, was perhaps the most brilliant scientist in all of Europe. The personal physician of King Charles I, he studied diligently under an anatomist colleague of Galileo's.[32] It was during this same era that Galileo himself was placed under house arrest for confirming Copernicus's theory of heliocentrism—that the earth revolves around the sun, and not the other way around. Harvey was one of the pioneering scientists that insisted on the scientific method, basing the analysis of his research on experimental evidence alone and taking nothing as a given. Prior to Harvey's revolutionary discoveries, the continent took the research of another scientist—Galen—as a given.

Galen called himself a philosopher and a physician. He posited a two-way circulatory system, with venous blood generating from the liver and arterial blood generating from the heart. The lungs played a role by releasing any waste material from the blood as soot into the air. Harvey relied exclusively on experimental evidence

---

32 Fjordman, "The Experimental Method and the Rise of Modern Science," *The Brussels Journal*, January 22, 2010, https://www.brusselsjournal.com/node/4285.

to determine otherwise—his conclusions were so precise that they remain essentially the same as what can be found in contemporary textbooks. However, when he published his findings, Harvey—the preeminent scientific mind of his era—was met with near-unanimous criticism.

In paving the way for modern experimental science, Harvey necessarily rejected two fundamental backbones of his culture: the church and the overreliance on rationalism. In regard to the former, Harvey steadfastly refused to attribute anything he could not prove to a great mystery of the divine cosmos. This alone put him at odds with many of his peers. In regard to the latter, Harvey refused to base his determinations on the power of thought alone—a strategy that was particularly *en vogue* at the time. If his results were true, the things he rejected in arriving at his conclusions were of the type that could cause an existential crisis in the scientific world. The uproar his research caused plagued him until his death in 1657. It wasn't until years later that the community and the culture writ large was able to adjust and evolve enough to embrace his findings.[33] Today, Harvey is considered the father of modern physiology—and his treatise remains one of the most significant of the modern scientific era.

In hindsight, a societal adjustment around how we view our circulatory system seems like nothing compared to the societal adjustment needed in order to embrace and create widespread knowledge about a biological system directly tied to one of the most taboo substances on the planet. The church and a rationalist approach to science represented two of the most commonly held belief systems in Harvey's time—and his research findings pushed back against them both. As

---

33   Kenneth E. Barber, "William Harvey and the Discovery of the Human Circulatory System," Encyclopedia.com, last updated March 21, 2020, https://www.encyclopedia.com/science/encyclopedias-almanacs-transcripts-and-maps/william-harvey-and-discovery-human-circulatory-system.

discussed in chapter 2, one of the greatest threats to our collective understanding and acceptance of cannabis as medicine is our society's commonly held belief that weed is bad. Understanding the leaf on its own is one means of slowly pushing back against the stereotype—but the endocannabinoid system and its incredible potential for healing the body is the ultimate trump card. Collectively understanding and accepting the uses of this bodily system has the power to put to rest all uniformly negative assumptions about cannabis.

So what is the endocannabinoid system—and what makes it so revolutionary?

UNDERSTANDING THE ENDOCANNABINOID SYSTEM

When you consume CBD oil sublingually, most of the substance gets taken up by a major artery found under the tongue, and the other part goes through a traditional edible route. The former is the most desired route and the reason it is instructed to hold the solution under your tongue for some number of seconds. It is a quicker route to absorption than getting metabolized through the stomach, and once in the bloodstream, CBD can readily cross the blood–brain barrier in its lipid nature. It is at this point that cannabinoid consumption can attach to processes that allow the receptors of the endocannabinoid system to go into action in the process of healing.

Our circulatory system's main instrument is the heart, made up of cardiac myocytes, fibroblasts, and other cells. The nervous system's main instruments are the brain and nerves themselves—and subsequently the neurons, glial cells, and neurotransmitters that give us our understanding of the world. The first thing that makes the endocannabinoid system so unique is that its main instruments, the cannabinoid receptors and the endocannabinoids that connect to them like a lock and key, are not found in just one location—rather, they are spread throughout the body. They're not tied to a single organ—yet they have a significant impact on several. The system's primary mode of operation can seem deceptively simple: resting like a sort of cellular net all across our internal organs, our cannabinoid receptors receive and process cannabinoids floating in our bloodstream. Those cannabinoids include endogenous cannabinoids—the ones our body produces naturally—and exogeneous cannabinoids, including phytocannabinoids, or cannabinoids that come from plants.

> Like a sort of cellular net all across our internal organs, our cannabinoid receptors receive and process cannabinoids floating in our bloodstream.

One of my favorite myths to debunk is the idea that all cannabinoids come from cannabis. That may be what the name suggests, but in fact, phytocannabinoids can be found in cacao, licorice, echinacea, electric daisy, Japanese liverwort, kava, black truffles, and many other plant species. This makes the intense regulatory framework around cannabis all the more mystifying, scientifically speaking—we can extract cannabinoids, including CBD, from plants that are perfectly legal, and when the compounds are isolate, they look exactly the same regardless of what plant they come from. Perhaps if this fact were more well known, regulators may take a more pragmatic approach.

The endocannabinoid system has been called "one of the most important physiologic systems involved in establishing and maintaining human health."[34] Endocannabinoids themselves have been called "arguably one of the most widespread and versatile signaling molecules known to man"[35] and "literally a bridge between the body and the mind."[36] And this bridge thus allows for heightened responses that will stimulate our overall lifestyle. The formation of Erykah Badu's band The Cannabinoids, for instance, is recognition of the power of the ECS, as her band is a "creation of music that affects the brain" and is meant to have the "audience feel the intensity of" her music.[37] The ECS has the power to stimulate our appetite or to take it away. It can relieve pain, nausea, and anxiety.

In my own son, I saw that it can relieve seizures and provide a balance, as I like to call it—it activates our body's own self-repair system. There's something powerful in this system—and yet despite the deceptively simple way it operates, because it is so

> This complex system modulates our body's homeostasis—without it, every other system in our body would be in danger of abnormalities. From head to toe, all of our systems are truly connected.

34   Hui-Chen Lu et al., "An introduction to the endogenous cannabinoid system," *Biological Psychiatry*, April 1, 2016; 79(7): 516–525, https://www.ncbi.nlm.nih.gov/pmc/articles/PMC4789136/.

35   "Human Endocannabinoid System," UCLA, accessed April 2020, https://www.uclahealth.org/cannabis/human-endocannabinoid-system.

36   Bradley E. Alger, "Getting High on the Endocannabinoid System, *Cerebrum*, November 1, 2013: 14, https://www.ncbi.nlm.nih.gov/pmc/articles/PMC3997295/.

37   "Interview: Erykah Badu Introduces Her Cannabis Crew," Complex, March 23, 2012, https://www.complex.com/music/2012/03/interview-erykah-badu-cannabinoids-sxsw.

multifaceted in nature, and touches upon so many different functions, this system can be hard to sum up. However there is a common link between each of these descriptions, and that's what ultimately defines the endocannabinoid system: millions of years old, and found in the bodies of every animal on earth, this complex system modulates our body's homeostasis—without it, every other system in our body would be in danger of abnormalities. From head to toe, all of our systems are truly connected.

The endocannabinoid system provides homeostasis by balancing and responding to the biological needs of our nervous system, internal organs, connective tissues, and immune system. It reads what our body needs to rebalance, and it triggers the right reactions to make that happen. This system impacts the entire body. Now, let's take a closer look at how this big-picture goal of homeostasis is actually made possible on a biological level.

A MESSENGER SYSTEM

The endocannabinoid system is, at its core, a messaging system—and in this single respect, it's not unique. In fact, it would be nearly impossible to write of the complex messaging mechanisms found within the endocannabinoid system without first considering its closely related cousin: the central nervous system.

The nervous system was first discovered, as so many others, by the ancient Greeks. Their logic mistakenly placed the heart as the system's center, from which all nerves stemmed. In the second century CE, Galen took another stab at the approach, more accurately suggesting the nerves stemmed from the brain. Galen's many successors understood that nerves were responsible for sensation, emotion, and possibly consciousness itself—in the eleventh century, the Islamic philosopher Avicenna wrote in his *Canon of Medicine* that "dryness in the nerves is the state which follows anger."[38] However, the scientific community remained unsure of the exact mechanism that allowed for communication of information within the nervous system—and they certainly didn't understand how that translated into things like moods and emotions.

It was not until the early twentieth century that a scientist named Santiago Ramón y Cajal discovered that mechanism—and his research paved the way for much of what we are able to understand about the brain and human psychology today. He discovered that neurons—or brain cells—communicate by sending chemical messengers—or neurotransmitters—to one another via cellular junctions called synapses. Ramón y Cajal dubbed the space between neurons, where the messages flow, the "synaptic cleft."

You can think of each neuron as a smartphone and the neurotransmitter as the text. A neuron that sends a neighboring neuron a neurotransmitter message is considered "presynaptic." The neuron that receives that text is considered "postsynaptic." What scientists did not discover until much later was that this neural transmission is not just a two-way conversation.

For decades, it was understood that the postsynaptic neurons exclusively receive information conveyed by neurotransmitters. As it turns out, they also sometimes forward information to a third party—and the third-party receptors aren't just located on the nearby neurons, although many certainly are. Rather, they are located throughout our entire bodies, waiting for an informative text from unique messenger chemicals that may act like neurotransmitters in some sense but are made up of an entirely different substance.

So what are these mysterious messengers? And what makes them so different from the neurotransmitters that they comprise an entirely different body system?

---

38   "A history of the nervous system," Stanford University, accessed April 2020, https://web.stanford.edu/class/history13/earlysciencelab/body/nervespages/nerves.html.

ENDOCANNABINOIDS

The chemical messengers sent from postsynaptic neurons to those mysterious third-party receptors are known as endogenously produced cannabinoids, or cannabinoids produced within our own bodies—endocannabinoids for short. Their strange retrograde motion—originating from the presynaptic rather than the postsynaptic neuron—is not the only thing that differentiates them from their neurotransmitter cousins, however. On a molecular level, neurotransmitters interact with nearby neurons by binding to specific receptor molecules on the cell's surface. Those receptors are made up of unique chemicals designed to react with the neurotransmitter and read its message.

Endocannabinoids are unique in their retrograde signaling—but they're diverse in other ways, too, including in their nonretrograde signaling (postsynaptic neurons activate postsynaptic CB1 receptors or transient receptor potential vanillioid-type 1 [TRPV1] channels and neuron-astrocyte endocannabinoid signaling).

Endocannabinoids, on the other hand, are lipids—and this is one of several reasons the endocannabinoid system is not just another, newer arm of our nervous system. Neuronal synapses simply don't have the right chemical makeup to read the lipid's message. So, the lipids go elsewhere—not just short distances within the brain, but into cells in our gut, our limbs, our musculature. In fact, lipids don't just go elsewhere: they go *everywhere*.[39] Therefore,

---

39   Bradley E. Alger, "Getting High on the Endocannabinoid System, *Cerebrum*, November 1, 2013: 14, https://www.ncbi.nlm.nih.gov/pmc/articles/PMC3997295/.

we now know that these receptors are the most diverse and versatile known to mankind.

The two most well-studied endocannabinoid ligands, or molecules, are N-arachidonyl-ethanolamide (anandamide or AEA) and sn-2-arachidonoyl-glycerol (2-AG). For our purposes, their names are not as important as their functionality—and their functionality begins by binding like a lock and key with their own, personalized receptors, which serve the singular purpose of reading the messages these endocannabinoids contain and putting them to use to restore balance within our system.

CANNABINOID RECEPTORS

Scientific research has a long way to go in terms of exploring our endocannabinoid system further. We currently know that cannabinoids can engage our bodies using various receptors, many of which we don't fully understand. The research will surely expand on this in upcoming years, and with that in mind, I'll keep the focus here on the two most well-known cannabinoid receptors: cannabinoid receptor type 1 (CB1) and cannabinoid receptor type 2 (CB2).[40] These receptors are both GPCRs, or G protein coupled receptors, which span the cell membrane activating processes intercellularly, and like an inbox they recognize and relay signaling across the cell membrane.

The first discovered cannabinoid receptor, CB1, is located primarily in the central nervous system, including the parts of our brains responsible for learning and memory, decision-making, emotional reactions, executive functioning—and sensory and motor responsiveness. Returning to the aforementioned purpose of the

---

40   Ibid, https://www.ncbi.nlm.nih.gov/pmc/articles/PMC3997295/.

endocannabinoid system, how might the receptors found within the brain specifically ensure homeostasis and balance? The answer lies somewhere in that three-way call between neurons. Exciting new research has found that, in receiving the endocannabinoid messages sent from the postsynaptic neuron, CB1 receptors can play a role in mitigating the messages neurons receive via neurotransmitter. Neurotransmitter messages can cause everything from stress to anxiety, from a sense of fear to a sense of hunger. That fact alone is a miracle of scientific research—but to consider that another bodily system could purposely alter those messages, either by exacerbating them or reducing them, is truly revolutionary, and raises meaningful questions about the nature of the mind and the body alike.[41]

CB2 receptors generally appear outside of the central nervous system. Present in our vascular system, microglia, spleens, tonsils, and throughout the gut, as well as in our brains, these receptors are generally associated with our immune and gastrointestinal systems.

With this new receptor, let's return again to the question of how receptors in these specific areas of our bodies might ensure homeostasis. To use the immune system and gastrointestinal system as primary examples, the answer seems quite apparent. Our immune system is charged with protecting us from disease and does so through a number of responses. If our body cannot return to a state of homeostasis after successfully implementing those responses, the consequences can be life-threatening over time, with chronic inflammation as just one example. CB2 receptors charged with restoring balance through the synthesis of cannabinoid molecules may well aid our immune system responses and restore functionality more readily. Chronic disorders of the gastrointestinal system are also caused by a body unable to bring itself back to balance. CB2 receptors located

---

41   Ibid, https://www.ncbi.nlm.nih.gov/pmc/articles/PMC3997295/.

here may offer the potential to restore healthy gut function—which in turn could offer relief for millions of suffering individuals.[42]

CANNABINOID SYNTHESIS: THE MISSING LINK

The third—and equally important—element of the endocannabinoid system are the enzymes responsible for the successful synthesis of the endocannabinoid into its dedicated receptor or the degradation of the endocannabinoid before the task can be implemented. The interactions between these three elements present truly endless possibilities for action within the system as a whole—and our challenge as researchers is to make sense of those possibilities as best as we can. In the meantime, I'll explain the basic mechanism of action caused by enzyme utilization—and then will pull the whole system together with two examples that will clarify some of the complexities outlined thus far.

Earlier, I mentioned that neuronal synapses don't have the right cellular makeup to read lipid-based cannabinoid messengers. Cannabinoid receptors, however, do have what it takes to read them—and enzymes guide that action. Enzymes are the fuel, the catalysts, the middlemen that drive these synapses. For instance, the endocannabinoid known as AEA can be synthesized from an enzyme known as hydrolyzed N-arachidonoylphosphatidylethanolamine, or NAPE. It can be degraded by an enzyme known as hydrolase (FAAH). The endocannabinoid 2-AG may be synthesized by an enzyme known as DAGL-alpha and degraded by

> Enzymes are the fuel, the catalysts, the middlemen that drive these synapses.

---

42   Amey Dhopeshwarkar et al., "CB2 Cannabinoid Receptors as a Therapeutic Target—What Does the Future Hold?," *Molecular Pharmacology*, October 2014; 86(4): 430–437, https://www.ncbi.nlm.nih.gov/pmc/articles/PMC4164977/.

enzymes MAGL, ABHD-6, and ABHD-12. In many instances, the inhibition of endocannabinoid degradation allows the endocannabinoid to be read, synthesized, and put to use in restoring homeostasis. In many other instances, when endocannabinoid degradation cannot be prevented, our body can suffer. This is just one example of how complex this signaling can be.

As our first example, let's take pain as just one of many intriguing instances of the receptor CB1's power to heal and restore our bodies. Endocannabinoids that react on CB1 receptors have been shown to have a mediatory effect on pain. However, if FAAH or other enzymes degrade the endocannabinoid first, there's less of an opportunity for that effect to take place. URB597 is a chemical compound that inhibits FAAH, and therefore makes the endocannabinoid AEA more active and available for synthesis. Inhibition of FAAH and MAGL specifically promote a reduction of both neuropathic and visceral pain mechanisms. This is an example of the ability to modulate through indirect targeting or upstream activity—not trying to target the endocannabinoid system directly but rather its environment. The possibilities for understanding in this space are incredible: if we could modulate pain, for instance, without the use of prescription medication like opioids, which present a high risk for addiction, how many lives might we save?

As a second example, let's consider what can happen when degradation is not prevented. In response to chronic stress, the brain sees a reduction in AEA levels, and therefore increased levels of the degradation enzyme FAAH. On the other hand, inhibitors of degradation enzymes of the endocannabinoid system can reduce stress. This may not seem like a major example—but the fact that we can map this as a possible mechanism for stress means that we have the potential to study it further and understand chronic stress and its possible cures better than ever before.

This general summary represents the very beginning of our insights into endocannabinoids, cannabinoid receptors, enzymes, and their complex interactions with each other and our other body systems. The research is young and the field wide open for promising exploration.

Equally open for exploration is the study of how exogenous cannabinoids factor into the endocannabinoid system. We have a very promising foundation to work from, and the direction we are headed points to an exciting and sophisticated future for cannabis medicine. Modulation of the endocannabinoid system is a target for therapeutic benefits. Understanding how to properly target the CB1 psychoactive receptor versus the CB2 receptor is key to this modulation. These examples and mechanistic understandings may strike you as better suited for medical or science textbooks—but bear with me: it is absolutely necessary to highlight what we know and what we don't know here so we can fill in the gaps of this industry.

EXOGENOUS CANNABINOIDS

Interestingly, science is starting to identify the internal mechanisms that the endocannabinoid system can influence. This will be helpful in providing new directions toward treatment of disease. Unfortunately, the bridge to gap is how the phytocannabinoids that come from plants specifically target these mechanisms. Now that we have a basis of understanding for the endocannabinoid system, we can begin to see THC, CBD, and other phytocannabinoids in a new, clearer way. For all the mysteries of the endocannabinoid system itself, the knowledge we now have about the way exogenous cannabinoids can interact with that system strips much of the mystery and mystique from the cannabis plant—and I consider that a great thing. Just the word "cannabis" being embedded in the endocannabinoid system may raise eyebrows and lead to doubts about the system itself. However, I've said it before and I'll say it again: knowledge is power, and the more we understand, the more able we are to collectively clarify the stereotypes.

Imagine for a moment a blood cell somehow naturally occurring in nature, outside of our own bodies, with a structure so similar to our own that when we ingest it, our bodies would not recognize the difference. What if all we had to do to build tone in our bodies was ingest a naturally occurring muscle cell? Sure, when we eat meat, we ingest protein, which is a building block for musculature. But the body does a lot of work in translating that protein into something it can use. Phytocannabinoids—those cannabinoids that occur in many different types of plants, including marijuana—are so similar in structure to our endogenous cannabinoids that some fit perfectly, like the lock and key, into currently identified receptors. Our bodies recognize the phytocannabinoids as a natural compound that chemically fit right into the processes of the endocannabinoid system.

Keeping in mind the numerous phytocannabinoids we don't yet understand, and those numerous receptors we have yet to discover in full, it's somewhat understandable that we don't have all the answers when it comes to how THC and CBD specifically interact with the endocannabinoid system. But how about the over five hundred molecules within the cannabis genus and over one hundred thirty cannabinoids alone that we have somewhat identified but have not characterized? How do they work when isolated? How do they work together? And how do we know that these interactions are beneficial?

We know that THC interacts primarily with the CB1 receptor, and we know that, somewhat beautifully, CBD does not significantly bind to either receptor but instead is an influencer of many processes or a guide. CBD can set into motion many different mechanisms that can influence the endocannabinoid system in balance and homeostasis of other bodily systems.

We don't have defined insight into how so many other phyto-cannabinoids process through our endocannabinoid system or, if inhaled—rather than ingested in a molecularly pure form—interact with the other elements of the plant itself, including the aromatic terpenes, flavonoids, pinenes, and other compounds numbering over five hundred different chemicals in total. Just as THC and CBD work so differently, the possibilities of the other cannabinoids are intriguing. Targeting the endocannabinoid system is like controlling the environment of a symptomatic condition or disease of any kind. It's the recognition that every component within our bodily systems is interconnected, and if we control the inflammation and acidity in the environment of the targeted diseased areas, we can target the ECS to control nearly any small symptom of any complex disease. We have empirical evidence of CBD's multitude of benefits—not only Macario's miraculous recovery, but also the benefits the compound has as an anti-inflammatory agent, an agent in providing gastrointestinal relief, and many others.

In 2017, the DEA made clear that any plant within the cannabis genus would remain as a Schedule 1 controlled substance. The research barriers, therefore, also remain in place. We have all of the blank pieces of the puzzle mapped out in front of us. We understand the leaf, we understand the basics of our unique bodily system that can process the compounds found within that leaf. Research, and research alone, can provide the missing links needed to clarify unanswered questions around THC, CBD, and other potentially powerful cannabinoids and how to best target the endocannabinoid system to restore balance.

Macario's life was changed thanks to the growing body of literature about the endocannabinoid system that caught my eye as I searched for anything that might help. It was changed thanks to the intriguing insights into how exogenous cannabinoids can help give our endocannabinoid system a jump-start, kicking it into action as it seeks out homeostasis. He's living proof of the incredible potential of this system—and I desperately want to see that potential blossom during my lifetime and his.

* * *

As I've continued my own research into cannabis and the endocannabinoid system, water often comes in handy as the perfect metaphor. When we drink water, our entire body becomes replenished. It's not just our chapped lips or our parched tongue—water moves through every part of us, restoring the parts that need it most. It's intuitive and adaptive. It's sensitive to the ever-changing inner circumstances of our biological makeup. It's not patterned or routine—rather, it's responsive. So, too, is the endocannabinoid system. Whether endogenous or exogenous, the cannabinoids that move through us have the capacity, often utilized, to replenish our system, providing slight adjustments here and there in aid of restoring an equilibrium, a peace throughout not just the body but the mind as well.

In Western medicine, we often veer away from the term "holistic." Medicine is supposed to target one thing, not several. And even with that being the goal, it never does. Clinical trials define side effects that extend beyond the targeted healing in a negative way. Most often, the side effects are worth it because the need for healing a more immediate area of attention is more important. Even then, there's no easy way for the medical community to open to the possibility of a medicine that works holistically with our bodies and may have numerous positive outcomes. Outside of the problem of the cannabis taboo, we are met with the bias against supplements that claim to do just that: heal holistically. But all medical revolutions take time—and all are accompanied by a collective shift in mindset. William Harvey, the discoverer of our circulatory system and pioneer of experimental practice, experienced it his lifetime; Galileo before him; Copernicus before him, and on the list goes.

It's time for our society to merge the beauty of what we've learned with the beauty that we've always known. The endocannabinoid system is the perfect target for a much-needed change in the way we define medicine, its limitations, and its possibilities. In the next chapter, we will begin to explore the structural problems within the industry itself that perpetuate the lack of open-mindedness when it comes to the topic of cannabis. We will also consider what a real change in mindset might look like—and what might change along with it.

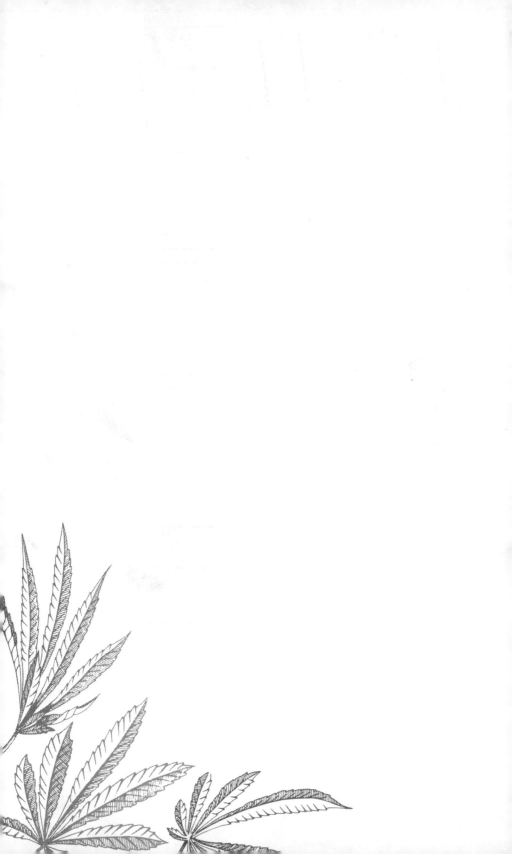

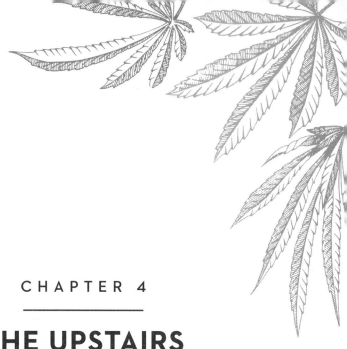

CHAPTER 4

THE UPSTAIRS DOWNSTAIRS EFFECT

L ife has a funny way of playing tricks on us. As soon as we think we've got it all figured out, that we have our futures planned with timelines and milestones pushing us toward success, it sends us untimely reminders of how little control we truly have in the cosmos. Rigidity rarely does us well in life—and clinging to certainty can leave us blind to the answers right in front of our noses. When the tide of life rolls in, we have two options: we can try desperately to protect our castles in the sand, or we can relax into the waves, trusting they'll take us to where we need to go.

In some ways, each and every one of us is a scientist: we spend thousands of hours inspecting our lives—past, present, and future— through a microscopic lens. We'd do well to become astronomers instead.

By zooming out that lens, we can begin to see where those crashing tides are taking us—and how they've prepared us for what's in store.

When I was in my twenties, I was no stranger to letting the waves take me where they would. I thought I was destined for professional basketball, but when Hurricane Katrina hit my Louisiana college town in 2005, plans changed. I was swept to a new shoreline. All the time and energy I'd spent building a promising basketball career were now focused on a new goal: becoming a doctor. I chose this route in part because of an innate passion for science and in part because I wanted my newborn daughter to have a mother who she saw as a role model and an inspiration someday down the road. So, I aspired to a medical degree at Georgetown University. Just two years later, however, a new tide pushed me toward a different path of becoming a cellular biologist. The story of why I shifted from medicine to biology, and the differences I observed between those two worlds once I did, forms the backbone of this chapter. I describe these differences as the Upstairs Downstairs effect—and these differences are impacting the world of cannabis in unexpected ways. We would do well to pay attention.

MY FATHER'S "MIRACLE"

During my second year at Georgetown, I got a call from my parents in Saskatchewan: my dad had been diagnosed with metastatic cancer of the esophagus. His doctors gave him less than three months to live. Over the phone, words like these can take some time to land. As I turned them over and over in my head, they just didn't connect. Terminal cancer? Says who? My father, gone from this world in a matter of months? I just didn't think it could happen. Some might call it denial—but deep in my bones I felt this was a tragedy that could be avoided.

I tell everyone that my dad isn't a man of few words—he's a man of none. Driven by a simple desire to see his family happy and provide them with whatever they may need, he's always silently made things happen behind the scenes, asking for no glory or praise in return. He supported my dreams since I was a child growing up in Canada—he even supported my dream of moving thousands of miles away to pursue my future. Hurricane Katrina had imprinted itself on my nervous system in such a way that when I heard my dad had just a few weeks longer to live, I didn't panic. I simply responded using the tools I had at my disposal. After all those years of my father supporting me, it was my turn to support him—and, along with the rest of my family, I sprang into action.

In some ways, I was in the right place at the right time to hear the news of my father. Studying at one of the country's most prestigious medical schools while having access to colleagues of the Washington Redskins gave me access to doctors at the top of their field. I asked my dad to fax me his medical record, confident that the experts I studied under could find some nuance in his diagnosis. My mentors examined my dad's CT scan and blood test results and came back to me with a simple message: drop everything and go home. My dad didn't have much time left.

I traveled back to Saskatchewan to be with my dad—but not to say goodbye. I arrived in my hometown ready to get to work. As it turned out, I wasn't the only one whose gut was telling me to remain optimistic, despite all evidence suggesting otherwise. My brother and mother felt the same way; importantly, Dad did too. Saskatchewan's indigenous roots run deep and infuse the culture in subtle yet meaningful ways. Thanks to the healing traditions and ancestral energy that continues to empower the tribal chiefs in the region, alternative medicine was embraced as a given much earlier than in many areas around the country and continent. These influences, as well as the spiritual influences of my Filipino family, meant we acknowledged a wider array of remedies than were on offer at the pharmacy. Set in this context, my father's diagnosis was not an ultimatum—rather, it was a bitter opportunity to take the holistic medicine practices in our roots and put them to work.

As I began poring over the annals of alternative medicine, I felt more and more hopeful. My dad was the one who instilled in me how powerful our beliefs can be in the pursuit of our dreams—and simply believing he could survive was 50 percent of the challenge. And he did believe. Over the course of the next month, we changed his diet, implemented supplementation, and walked every day with him. Dad drank beet juice, ate every blackberry he could get his hands on, and tasted enough honey to quench the cravings of the biggest sweet tooth. The doctors had told my father he had less than three months to live. Just two months after that diagnosis, he was cancer free.

Because his miraculous recovery seemed systematically impossible, they called my dad a miracle. But I began to wonder: how many more people would be considered a miracle if we allowed ourselves to stretch the limits of what we thought was possible? My dad's recovery taught me an important lesson: the protocols and systems that are put into place, that serve as guidelines in the medical world, are not a straight line. Our bodies have the ability to self-repair and to fight—and sometimes we can't always explain why. But that doesn't mean we shouldn't try.

It wasn't enough to call it a miracle. I wanted to understand the mechanism of action behind my father's cure—and I

> **Our bodies have the ability to self-repair and to fight— and sometimes we can't always explain why. But that doesn't mean we shouldn't try.**

realized if there was any chance in explaining what happened to my dad, I wasn't going to learn it in medical school. Abnormalities like my father's cancer occur on a molecular level in the body, as does any possible treatment for those abnormalities. Medicine is the practice of implementing what has already been researched and created. I no longer wanted to be the practitioner—I wanted to be the philosopher.

MD TO PhD

Transitioning from a path toward an MD to a PhD would allow me to examine abnormalities at their root. I started a PhD program at Georgetown's neuroscience department before transferring to a program in Nashville at Vanderbilt. In some ways, the years that followed were some of the hardest in my life. Vanderbilt is a demanding institution, and with two young children at home it was hard to focus on my thesis and my thesis alone—but I made it work. And it wasn't long into my program that I began to realize my background and experience gave me a unique perspective on the petri dishes and lab experiments before me.

In the years spent working to obtain my PhD, I was particularly interested in genetic factors that mimicked offset effects of certain chemotherapies leading to cardiotoxicity and thus malformations in the heart—and ultimately heart disease. I looked at every cell type in isolation, from frozen tissue in a diseased state to living cells in various environments, studying them closely under my microscope. Over the course of my research, I ultimately developed an important protocol at Vanderbilt in which I successfully isolated a mouse cardiomyocyte— the cardiac cells that keep the heart beating. It felt good to contribute something big to my research university, but in the process, I learned a lesson far more basic and essential.

I learned the body never operates in a straight line. Even the slightest difference in process can make a difference between a detrimental or "miraculous" result. This lesson, paired with the lessons from my dad's recovery from terminal cancer, gripped me to my core. I'd seen how doctors work and operate during my time shadowing numerous medical professionals of all different types. I'd seen how scientists work and operate during my time obtaining my PhD. But what stuck with me most was the intersection of these two worlds: my dad. The patient. The humans ultimately impacted by a doctor's expertise and a scientist's discoveries.

Toward the end of my thesis, I became drawn to translational biology, an emerging field of practice focused on bringing exciting new research more easily from the lab to the patient and his or her treatment—from bench to bedside, as it is colloquially put. It seemed clear to me that precision medicine, or treatment based on a patient's specific personalized needs, was the future—and if precision medicine was the goal, translational biology seemed to be a clear path to getting there. But translational biology relies on a symbiosis between the scientific and medical fields. And the frank reality of these worlds is that they often feel mutually exclusive.

THE UPSTAIRS DOWNSTAIRS EFFECT: THE PROBLEM

As a scientist, I walked into the cancer center that patients came to for their testing and treatments every day. The main floor held the waiting room and treatment room for the patients. The elevators on the right led to the oncologists' offices. The elevators to the left led to the science labs. I can count on one hand the number of times I went to the oncology offices, and the only time I went through the patient treatment rooms was to take a shortcut to another medical research building. In fact, I did not know a single name of any of the oncologists that worked in the same building as me. We scientists were upstairs in our labs researching and creating data analysis, and the doctors were downstairs interacting with patients. We hardly ever communicated with doctors—and never communicated with the patients themselves.

When it came time to get a scientific understanding of Macario's treatment—or even Dad's diagnosis—there were too many floors between where the treatment occurred and where the rationale for treatment originated, and where a more personalized treatment would lie. Many academic institutions have attempted to address this major gap in knowledge

> **We hardly ever communicated with doctors—and never communicated with the patients themselves.**

sharing by bringing scientists into rounds with doctors and coordinating luncheons where scientists could share their latest findings. I witnessed these efforts—and also, sadly, witnessed why so frequently nothing ever came from them. The Upstairs Downstairs effect may be seriously inhibiting novel discoveries and methods from arising—and, as we shall see, this has a significant impact on the world of medical cannabis, both now and in terms of what's possible for the future.

THE UPSTAIRS

At Vanderbilt, I found it temptingly easy to get sucked into the microscopic world beneath my lens—and I am certainly not the only one who did. This is the work and world of a biologist: you can isolate a single cell in a petri dish and study the exact same concept for years, yet still have more to learn. A side effect of becoming singularly focused on what lies between the fragile walls of a cell structure is that you can forget the cell type you're studying is one of hundreds that exist in the human body. You can forget that beyond your microscope, there are other scientists studying other types of cells, and that your work may interact and overlap with theirs in significant ways you're unable to see unless you zoom out the lens.

The way our current research landscape is structured, scientists spend years researching and writing papers with very specific insights that may never see the light of day or make an immediate difference in patients' lives. There are some heavy collaborative efforts, but generally there is somewhat of a lack of communication between researchers, and this leads to a net loss of knowledge that could change the way we think of our well-being and health. It is true that decades of research on a single cell can lead to incredible lifesaving discoveries. It is also true that biologists simply don't talk to each other as much as they should. As a group, we would do well to remember that discoveries can also be found by spontaneous interactions and chance encounters. Because we are siloed in our separate corridors in our research institutions, the possibility of those chance encounters is inherently limited. What are we missing?

When I was working on completing my thesis, I considered these issues—and yet because of time constraints I was unable to think too deeply about how they could be addressed. I was too focused on completing my paper or gathering more molecular data to prove my scientific claim so that my principal investigator could reapply for a grant. I knew a change needed to happen in the field, but I was far too consumed with problems in the here and now to be considering long-term issues that verged on the philosophical. Between seminars, meetings, and experiments, there was hardly enough time to perform the analyses needed—and what time I did have was spent on raising my toddlers. Siloed corridors, time constraints, and more—and those are just the concerns happening upstairs in the labs. Downstairs, in the medical hallways, doctors faced problems of their own.

THE DOWNSTAIRS

If the upstairs part of the problem lies in the limited interaction between various types of scientists—chemists, pharmacologists, biologists all included—in the research labs, whose work could be informing and building off one another's, the downstairs part of the problem lies in the chaotic hospital floor. There is not just one but many layers of problems with the way our current medical landscape is structured. Anyone who has ever been to a doctor's office can attest to the utter lack of time on a medical practitioner's hands on any given day. Primary care physicians often see up to twenty patients a day[43] and work an average of fifty-one hours a week. With what extra time might physicians work with scientists to determine novel solutions for their patients? And even if they had the time, it's not a straightforward answer as to whether those novel solutions would be admissible. Doctors are beholden to the rules and protocols of the institutions they work for. No matter which way you cut it, change comes slowly in the medical world.

Even if scientists and doctors had the time, there is simply no straightforward pathway for knowledge sharing between what insights come about upstairs and what might get translated directly to a patient downstairs. To extend the metaphor, we have many floors between these departments, but we seem to be lacking a dedicated stairwell. Entrenched medical protocols and the inability of the focused scientist

---

43 "2018 Survey of America's Physicians," Physicians Foundation, last updated September 2018, https://physiciansfoundation.org/wp-content/uploads/2018/09/physicians-survey-results-final-2018.pdf.

to translate their research into existing problems may both contribute to the problem, but ultimately there's nobody to blame. Do scientists need to think more like physicians and physicians more like scientists? Is there enough time for either? Does there need to be a dedicated buffer professional—a physician scientist—who can help bridge the gap between upstairs and downstairs? It is true that institutions are trying to provide that buffer by utilizing their patient data and publishing it in order to come up with more real-time solutions—but can't the science be used more efficiently? Can't the communication between scientist and physician be more productive than a free lunch on an interesting topic?

* * *

The Upstairs Downstairs effect is, at its foundation, a fundamental problem of a lack of communication between two related but disparate fields of study and practice.

The Upstairs Downstairs effect is, at its foundation, a fundamental problem of a lack of communication between two related but disparate fields of study and practice. But that communication breakdown is not necessarily industry specific. Contemporary society as a whole has a proclivity to categorize, define, and draw boundaries, rules, and restrictions—yet when we do this, we may be missing out on emergent systems, emergent paths to knowledge, chance encounters, spontaneous discoveries, serendipity, fate. Life is far more interconnected than it may seem, and the rigid boundaries we draw are much more fluid, whether we like it or not—the self-healing benefits of the endocannabinoid system is the perfect example of this interconnectedness within our own bodies. Now that we've determined a challenge in the medical and biological world, let's examine the direct impacts this has on the world of cannabis.

CANNABIS AND THE UPSTAIRS DOWNSTAIRS EFFECT

When you're walking down the over-the-counter medicine aisle at the grocery store, nearly every medication or supplement you see originally came from a plant. To translate a plant into a medicine, scientists use developmental molecular biology to individually isolate the plant's molecules and reagents. The substance is then subject to years and years of benchwork testing before scientists create the final product. The end result—the medicine—then undergoes rigorous clinical phase trials testing at a cost of millions of dollars. It's tested on animals, then humans, in order to reach eventual FDA approval. Now, we know from chapter 3 that there are significant barriers to researching cannabis—even though the plant has been used medicinally for thousands of years. We now also know that the Upstairs Downstairs effect can make it exceedingly difficult for medical research to get translated to patient treatments. It can take years to research and write a single medical paper, and it can take years to change protocols at medical institutions. Why, then, does it seem like the cannabis industry has turned these truths on their heads?

WHERE IS THE RESEARCH?

In the traditional order of things, the wait for medical claims to translate into prescriptions or altered protocols can be almost excruciating. Yet, in the realm of cannabis, we seem to be rushing toward translational biology at an increasingly dangerous pace. If the Upstairs Downstairs effect demonstrates the consequences of medicine and research moving too slowly, the cannabis space certainly sits at the opposite end of the spectrum, demonstrating the consequences of claims and conclusions being publicized and promoted way before the data and research prove them out.

I saw this issue firsthand when I was looking for an alternative treatment for Macario. Cannabis was so widespread on the market that I intuited there must be at least some research to back up the incredible claims of this plant. And yet when I searched for this type of research, there was none. In the three years since then, billions of dollars have been dumped into the cannabis industry—and there is still no significant new research. Not anything complete. Instead, the industry relies primarily on anecdotal stories for its success. I read through many of these myself as I became familiarized with the various claims of cannabis and CBD. But when it came to treating my son, I needed something more than a story. My child was sick, and I couldn't rely on anecdotal claims alone—especially when the claims themselves were at times as inconsistent as the products I was testing. At times, it felt like I was wandering through a funhouse, where every time I tried to orient myself, a trick mirror pointed me in a different direction. There was no foundational evidence, no consistent product, and above all, no clarity.

CANNABIS IS MORE THAN ENTERTAINMENT

Since 2018, CBD has exploded onto the marketplace at a rate nobody could've predicted even five years ago—and both the scientific and medical realms are finding themselves in a bind. Still limited by restrictions on research, scientists are struggling to gather data and engage in testing that will take years to form into a truly meaningful body of research, a canon from which stable cannabis medicines can arise—but their numbers are few. Meanwhile, doctors are seeing patients like a revolving door and few are eager to jump on the medical marijuana bandwagon.

Despite needing more than just anecdotes, I realize my own son provides anecdotal evidence of a sort for the power of CBD and medical cannabis more generally. And while the anecdotes may not equate scientific rigor, they can be used for something useful: taken as a whole and placed in the larger context of the history of the plant, it is clear cannabis is a powerful medicine with healing properties of which we are only beginning to realize the full extent. So why have we allowed a powerful substance to slip through the rigors of testing and research and flood the market with unsubstantiated claims? Why have we ceded control of cannabis to the realm of entertainment and consumer marketing?

The hesitation of doctors and scientists alike to enter the cannabis space is indicative of yet another layer of obfuscation within the cannabis industry in general and in the medical and scientific professions writ large. In addition to the Upstairs Downstairs divide, there is another meaningful divide cannabis finds itself at the center of: the divide between holistic medicine and Western or modern medicine.

HOLISTIC MEDICINE VERSUS MODERN MEDICINE

When I read through the success stories about cannabis and CBD, I noticed an interesting thread that ran through each of them: as adamant as they were about what cannabis did for them, they were just as adamant that the world of science would never bother proving them. For many cannabis reviewers, it just didn't matter whether or not science backed their claims—and upon reflection, I could understand where they were coming from.

When I describe the Upstairs Downstairs effect, I'm specifically describing a problem that exists in modern Western medicine. In this world, descriptive claims may be a starting point, but on their own, they're not enough. When my father had cancer, I craved clarity about not just the how but the why—the world of science and research seeks to understand the mechanisms of action behind the claim, and it was for this reason I chose to join their ranks. It seeks to understand the inner workings of a cure or a disease and to replicate its findings on a broad scale, so that not just one individual can benefit but millions. These explorations take years, or decades, to confirm. Thus, a claim is not the end point but the beginning—from there, a scientist searches for answers through the scientific method, again, again, and yet again. The researchers upstairs work to find answers, and the medical professionals downstairs administer them once they're found. There may be a communication breakdown between them, but the two professions are at baseline working under the same umbrella—and that umbrella is modern medicine.

Before there was technology and testing and sterile labs, there were localized healers in every civilization across the globe, searching for and serving remedies, tonics, and yes—cures. Long before there were scientists studying disease at the level of a cell, these practitioners believed health lay not just in a single region of the body but rather in the harmony between mind, body, and spirit. Therein lies the primary challenge for the Western medical practitioner: in terms of measurement, the body itself is hardly a sum of all its parts. It presents enough challenges for variability and control in experimentation. But the mind and the spirit? Those expand far beyond the quantitative.

They are qualitative elements of health without boundaries or borders, uncontainable by the categories we try to place things neatly within. Holistic medicine acknowledges the interplay between mind, body, and spirit and works within that system, rather than outside of it. This system is far more descriptive than prescriptive—thus, by its very definition, holistic medicine seems to fall outside the purview of what Western science thinks it can touch. How did this happen— and how might the study of cannabis realign the tension between holistic/modern practices to be more integrated and perhaps even more cooperative?

THE HISTORY OF THE HOLISTIC/ MODERN MEDICINE DICHOTOMY

The dichotomy of holistic and modern medical practices was perhaps introduced by the man who is considered the father of Western medicine—the Greek physician Hippocrates. In his era, most medical practitioners attributed disease to spiritual or supernatural causes. As just one example, seizures like the one my son experienced in his earliest days were thought by the Greeks to be the consequence of angering the gods.[44] In 400 BCE, Hippocrates proposed something radically different—that diseases were born entirely by the body. In fact, his treatise *On the Sacred Disease* opens with a line describing epilepsy as "nowise more divine nor more sacred than other diseases, but as a natural cause from which it originates like other affections." The Hippocratic physicians drew connections between mind and body but did away with spiritual affectations in medicine.

Hundreds of years later, in the sixteenth century, a physician named Andreas Vesalius was granted permission to dissect the bodies of executed criminals. His seminal book on the human body—*On the Fabric of the Human Body*—justifiably cemented his reputation

---

44   Sneha Mantri, "Holistic Medicine and the Western Medical Tradition," *AMA Journal of Ethics*, March 2008, https://journalofethics.ama-assn.org/article/ holistic-medicine-and-western-medical-tradition/2008-03.

in the medical world as the father of modern anatomy. With this work, medicine essentially did away with the mind–body connection and focused entirely on the physical. The invention of the microscope made medicine even more specific and specialized—describing ailments of the body down to the level of the cell.

Western medicine began as an all-encompassing, holistic, mind–body–spirit practice. But slowly, over the course of hundreds of years, the introduction of specialized tools and a body-centered framework took the holistic practice of medicine and broke it down into a million fragmented pieces. Now you have scientists at the same institution siloed in different labs, peering through their microscopes at fractions of fractions of a human body—specific cells within organs that operate within body systems that, yes, eventually comprise a whole.

> If their work and treatment is like a dart hitting a bull's-eye on a board, holistic practices seem more like a slot machine. You might hit the jackpot—but you'll never know why.

This specialized culture has taken precedent in our culture, and it is easy to understand why, once a scientist is able to view such a distinct and singular entity as a cell in such incredible detail, holistic cures seem far too imprecise. If their work and treatment is like a dart hitting a bull's-eye on a board, holistic practices seem more like a slot machine. You might hit the jackpot—but you'll never know why.

CAN HOLISTIC AND WESTERN MEDICINE WORK TOGETHER?

Western medical practitioners are trained to view holistic medicine with a skeptic's eye—and contemporary holistic practitioners view the medical world in much the same way. The medical world is embedded with protocol, and specialization leads to critical integrative knowledge falling through the cracks. The holistic world is unregulated, and efficacy of supplements are wildly varied—as I found in my own experience testing CBD oils in the lab. Just as cannabis sits at the intersection between upstairs and downstairs, it also sits at the intersection between Western medicine and holistic practice. Both entities now prescribe cannabis—yet both are missing out on the full potential of this substance, because both are too committed to staying in their own lanes.

Both worlds have something to learn from each other. What would happen if we brought the modern technology utilized in the medical labs to the realm of holistic medicine? What if nonprescription holistic remedies could reliably bolster the health of those who take them? Neither my father nor my son would be here today if it wasn't for the strategic use of both modern and alternative medicine. But I had to figure out the right combination of both entirely on my own—and I had to create my own CBD precisely because this substance has one foot in both doors and is not being utilized to its full potential in either.

Cannabis has long been used as a medicine in holistic health practices, but the variability of potencies and effects make it hard to reliably administer. "Pot doctors," however, are trying to do just that, while many other doctors steer clear, reinforcing the stigma of the plant and its medical administration. Meanwhile, the science behind cannabis and its potential is not coming out nearly as quickly as the medicine itself—and all of these factors, taken as a whole, are rapidly overtaking any chance cannabis has to regain legitimacy. We need to change the industry before it's too late—but the question remains as to how we can do so.

TRANSLATIONAL BIOLOGY

In ancient cultures, there was often a point person in every village that individuals could turn to for medical needs. Now, understanding health and medical claims has become increasingly decentralized—and nowhere is this more true than in the world of cannabis. Because of a lack of consensus and scientific rigor, people are turning to online forums to get a better understanding of what certain cannabis strains and products can be used for what ailments, and almost none of it is rooted in clear understanding. Adding to the confusion is the actual sale of cannabis products themselves. I've seen CBD being sold everywhere from liquor stores to pharmacies—and being sold in everything from fancy chocolates to cups of coffee.

Even with large amounts of money being put into this space, there is hardly any money going toward actual research—and the research that needs to be done still falls under limiting federal regulations. Scientific study is slow going, and it seems funding that could be invested in long-term research is being diverted to products that can make a quick buck—CBD-infused ice cream and the like. Meanwhile, a whole class of individuals—and children like Macario—who could gain so much from a trusted cannabis medicine are suffering.

So how do we as a culture remedy this complex issue? If science moves slowly and the commercial sale of cannabis is moving increasingly quickly, is it even possible for cannabis and CBD to gain legitimacy in the medical world? I believe it is possible—and I believe translational biology may be the answer. The market seems to be in a place ready for transparency and education, but do we know what type of research needs to be done?

WHAT IS TRANSLATIONAL RESEARCH?

Translational research practices offer a multidisciplinary approach to medicine with the ultimate goal of improving health outcomes of the patient. This is a different approach to research being conducted in many labs today, which often focuses on developing understanding of a specific part of human mechanism and disease without looking at the body as the ultimate sum of its parts. This research is certainly important—but I believe a translational practice bridges the divide between upstairs and downstairs by giving doctors more to work with and bridges the divide between holistic and modern medicine by offering a more integrated approach.

*　*　*

If cannabis could be studied through a translational lens, with research being developed with the patient's needs in mind and outcomes being passed more quickly to doctors who could administer treatment accordingly to their patients, perhaps this plant would more quickly come into its own in the world of medicine. If we brought our highly sophisticated scientific tools to study ancient medicines that have existed for millennia, we could more easily combine the descriptive claims we've always known with the scientific rigor we have access to today. And most importantly, if scientists worked more closely with healthcare practitioners, the future of cannabis medicine would look a lot brighter. Unfortunately, it's not as easy as it sounds, but we can't fix something that we can't identify.

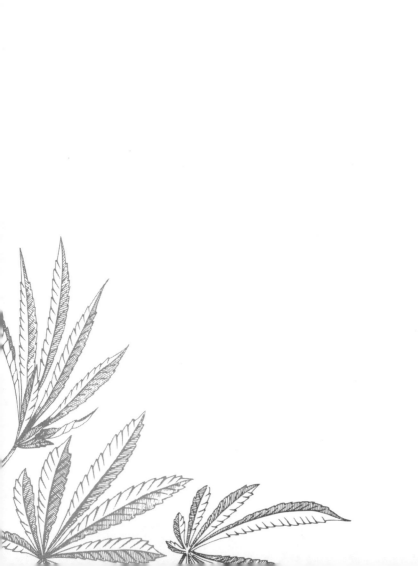

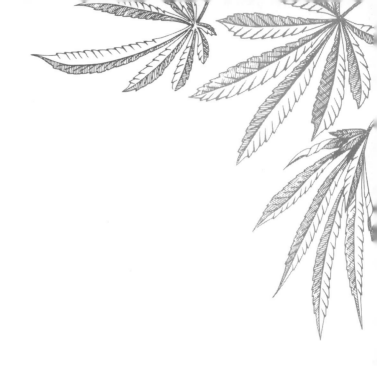

PART TWO

THE FUTURE OF CANNABIS

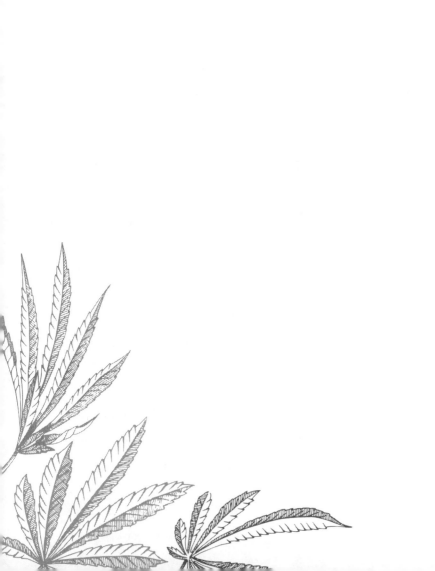

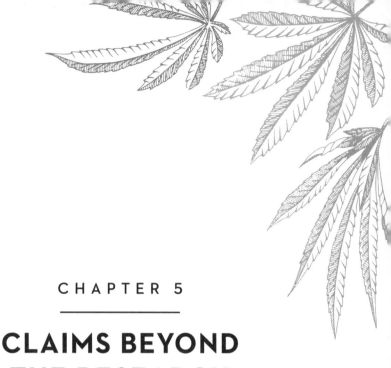

CHAPTER 5

CLAIMS BEYOND
THE RESEARCH

My professional origins as a medical-student-turned-PhD-student primed me to pick up on the connections—or lack thereof—between the two worlds. Over and over during my time as a student, I'd make a mental note of the siloed nature of both the hospital floor and the labs upstairs. Likewise, my father's illness primed me to pick up on a similar disconnect between holistic medical knowledge—the knowledge that saved my dad—and Western medical practice—the practice that felt more comfortable attributing my father's recovery from stage IV cancer to a miracle than to traditional, nonprescription remedies that remain stubbornly untested by scientific rigor. But it was another element of my life that primed me for an equally important personal and professional revelation—one I'd run into over and over again in my study and development of a cannabis product capable of saving my son.

My journey toward a PhD was much more than I could have ever bargained for. If I knew it would take as long as it did and create as many sleepless nights as it did, perhaps I wouldn't have pursued it. Even my mentors warned me my journey toward a PhD would be arduous at best. Their concern was simple enough: by the time I'd become a PhD candidate, I was a divorced mother of two toddlers. I worked harder than I thought possible in those years—and while juggling the responsibilities of motherhood and my professional ambition was strenuous and at times overwhelming, the balance of both roles enabled me to look at elements of the clinical world with a wider lens. In a sense, the responsibilities of being a mother to two young children instilled in me a more pragmatic viewpoint in every other facet of my life. It primed me to pick up on the realities—and inefficiencies—of drug discovery and development. Years later, it would help me discover how these inefficiencies relate to the cannabis industry—and why it's more important than ever to find a new route of research and reclaim the narrative about this plant.

The responsibilities of being a mother to two young children instilled in me a more pragmatic viewpoint in every other facet of my life.

As we've seen throughout this book, cannabis has incredible medicinal qualities—and they deserve to be properly researched so we can understand the full extent of its benefits. But because of its complex history, cannabis is already on the market, and individuals are already making claims about its medicinal value. In chapter 4, I discussed the complexities of the medical culture writ large, which make it difficult for cannabis to be taken seriously as a medicine. In this chapter, I want to explore the culture of medicine itself.

In exploring the complex path that must be followed for a claim or an idea to become proven medicine, I hope to underscore the significant fallibility in current claims being made about cannabis, both positive and negative. Despite the complexities we'll dig into in this chapter, the bottom line is clear: the research should move faster, and the claims individuals make about the plant should come far slower. Somewhere in the balance between the claims and the research, the truth about cannabis will be uncovered. Seeking it out sooner rather than later could change the culture and improve the quality of countless lives.

PLANT TO MEDICINE

Across cultures, eras, and civilizations, the goal of medicine has remained more or less the same: to relieve pain, to enable health, and to cure or prevent disease wherever possible. Achieving these aims requires determining a problem (a diagnosis) and administering a solution (a prescription). Thanks to modern technology and sophisticated medical imaging tools, diagnosing a medical problem in a patient has become a somewhat easier task than it once was—but the act of prescribing a solution that neatly addresses the diagnosis, while simple on its face, is in fact the culmination of years of research, billions of dollars, and multiple tests and approvals administered by multiple organizations and entities. More and more individuals are open to considering cannabis as a medicine—but what does it actually take for a plant to become a medicine, and what are the implications for the future of cannabis?

A SHORT HISTORY OF PHARMACOLOGY

For millennia, medicine originated in the soil—in the roots of plants, the bark of a tree, or the mold growing on rotting leaves or fruits. The prescription drugs of our ancestors were likely discovered through trial-and-error experimentation and careful observation over a stretch of time.[45] From plant to mouth, the process of discovering a medicine and administering it as a solution for a patient's particular diagnosis had a far less complex timeline and a far less time-consuming one as well.

In the eighteenth and nineteenth centuries, this straightforward administration of medication was underscored by the popular theory that organic compounds comprising living substances like plants contained a vital force that could not be created in the lab—meaning that medication would always need to come from the plant itself, rather than an inorganic, or nonliving, compound. In 1828, the chemist Friedrich Wöhler disproved this theory by creating urea, an organic compound, from ammonia, an inorganic compound.[46] In doing so, Wöhler became a founding figure and pioneer in the field of organic chemistry—and paved the way for modern pharmacology in the process.

The ability to create organic compounds from inorganic materials meant scientists could isolate the healing chemicals in the plants used for medicine and synthesize them in the lab—and eventually discover novel compounds under the microscope. Many modern medicines have their origins in this era, when plant-based remedies informed the rooms of budding pharmacology labs. Aspirin, first extracted from the bark of a willow tree, made its debut in the early twentieth century. And in 1928, a century after Wöhler's critical discovery, a biologist

---

45   "History of drug discovery and development," UCDavis, accessed April 2020, http:// scalettar.physics.ucdavis.edu/frs/historyofdrugdiscovery1.pdf.

46   "Friedrich Wöhler biography," Britannica, last updated May 2019, https://www.britannica.com/biography/Friedrich-Wohler.

named Alexander Fleming made an accidental discovery of his own when he noticed a blob of mold on one of his petri dishes was killing off a bacteria he was studying. Fleming's discovery was penicillin—the world's first true modern antibiotic. Two scientists, Howard Florey and Ernst Chain, scaled up the production of penicillin during World War II and saved millions of lives in the process. The mass production of this new "wonder drug"[47] became another crucial step toward the practice of modern medicine as we know it today.

Taken together, these milestones are important building blocks comprising the foundation of drug discovery and modern pharmacology. I share this consolidated history with you to illustrate both the primacy of plants in the medical labs when the field of drug discovery first came about and the recency of the field itself. It was not so long ago that plants were our primary form of medicine. Now, an entire framework exists to guide the discovery of a medicine—whether in a plant or elsewhere—to its ultimate culmination in your pillbox.

DRUG DISCOVERY

The discovery and development of new drugs was once firmly in the realm of the physician scientists—but in the second half of the twentieth century, one field diverged into two, and the separate domains of scientific research and clinical practice emerged.[48] The responsibility of drug discovery now falls to several distinct yet overlapping organizations, including academic institutions like the ones I worked for during my

---

47 "American Chemical Society National Historic Chemical Landmarks, Penicillin Production through Deep Tank Fermentation," American Chemical Society, accessed April 2020, https://www.acs.org/content/acs/en/education/whatischemistry/landmarks/penicillin.html.

48 C. Simone Fishburn, "Translational research: The changing landscape of drug discovery," *Drug Discovery Today* December 2012, http://www.ucdenver.edu/academics/colleges/pharmacy/Resources/Faculty/Documents/Retreat/Fishburn Translational Research Article 010413.pdf.

PhD candidacy, biotech companies, pharmaceutical companies, and the National Institutes of Health. If the upstairs/downstairs dichotomy has led to hampered communication between scientists and clinicians, the numerous parties involved in drug formulation has led to an even more complex tangle of communications, needs, and motivations—and much can get lost in translation.

Ideas for new drugs are most commonly formed in academia or biotech, but pharmaceutical companies are needed for funding, especially in the late stages of medicine development. The necessity of multiple parties' involvement in the creation of a single drug has led to a disjointed process of drug development. One academic paper on the topic describes the problem this way:

> *Several studies of drug development have shown large pharmaceutical companies don't serve as fertile grounds for innovation and are dependent on academics and biotech for fueling their pipeline. On the other hand, discovery scientists in academia or small biotech companies are often not trained in clinical considerations or business strategies and have little access to the necessary funding for proof of principle data needed to attract investment. Lack of communication between these parties has resulted in many good ideas lying unexploited, while many drug pipelines become barren.*[49]

Inefficiencies and complications aside, drug discovery and development generally follows a well-trodden trajectory, comprised of a series of steps. It doesn't always work this way—but this is the standard process:[50]

---

49 Ibid, http://www.ucdenver.edu/academics/colleges/pharmacy/Resources/Faculty/Documents/Retreat/Fishburn Translational Research Article 010413.pdf.

50 Compound Interest, "Understanding the drug discovery process," *Compound Chemical*, January 16, 2016, https://www.compoundchem.com/2016/01/16/drug-discovery/.

CLAIMS BEYOND THE RESEARCH

First, a target for drug discovery is identified—this is most often a biological mechanism involved in a disease. From there, scientists begin to test anywhere from five to ten thousand different molecules to understand how each interacts with that mechanism. This process of baseline drug discovery can take anywhere from three to five years, even longer depending on the mechanism.

From the thousands of compounds tested against the target, around two hundred fifty compounds will undergo preclinical trials to determine basic safety and how that compound behaves in a living organism. In vitro and in vivo testing are both used—the former involves testing molecules outside of a biological surrounding and the latter involves testing on animals, often rodents. This phase of testing can last up to two years.

Next, a compound undergoes three phases of clinical trials, in which it is tested on humans to ensure safety and efficacy. The first phase involves a small number of participants, to test dosing and to learn of any serious side effects. The second phase involves a larger number of participants, generally several hundred, and often compares the drug to a placebo. The third phase involves several thousand participants and large-scale monitoring of safety. Each of these trials is repeated many times. The FDA estimates that 70 percent of drugs make it through phase one testing, only a third pass through to phase two, and just 25–30 percent of the remaining get through phase three.[51] Overall, these three phases of testing can take six to seven years to complete.

Last, the FDA itself reviews all of the data and makes a decision whether or not to approve the drug. The approval period can take

---

51   "Drug discovery and development timeline," Researchgate, accessed April 2020, https://www.researchgate.net/figure/Drug-discovery-and-development-timeline-The-current-drug-approval-pipeline-can-take-15_fig1_308045230.

117

one to two years. Many other countries generally take the same route as the US FDA.

From discovery to approval, the development of a drug takes fifteen years on average, at an average cost of $2.5 billion.[52] And from all that research and development, the FDA approves an incredibly small number of drugs each year. In the early aughts, that number ranged in the midtwenties. In 2018, a record-setting fifty-nine drugs were approved by the organization—but even that represents a diminishingly small number of new medicines compared to the depth and breadth of research occurring behind the scenes.

> **From discovery to approval, the development of a drug takes fifteen years on average, at an average cost of $2.5 billion.**

Drug discovery often begins to meet a demand on the market—that is, a distinguishable diagnostic target for which to apply a drug. Other times, when there is not a demand, scientists are simply working in the lab and can build out a body of research on molecules or compounds that can be tapped into once a demand necessitates it. Cannabis studies don't fit neatly into either of these categories: because of federal restrictions on research of the plant, scientists don't have the opportunity to explore the compounds freely in the lab—and this baseline lack of understanding perpetuates lack of understanding about what demand the molecular compounds found in cannabis could possibly target.

---

52   Rick Mullin, "Cost to develop new pharmaceutical drug now exceeds $2.5B," *Chemical and Engineering News*, November 24, 2014, https://www.scientificameri-can.com/article/cost-to-develop-new-pharmaceutical-drug-now-exceeds-2-5b/.

HOW DOES THIS IMPACT CANNABIS?

The process of drug development and discovery costs billions of dollars and takes years, if not decades. Without a known target, scientists can explore the different functionalities of different molecules in the lab for an entire lifetime and still not know the full extent of those molecules' capabilities. As discussed in chapter 4, translational research could certainly help in cutting down the inefficiencies and possibly some of the expenses of this long development time. But even translational research requires rigorous testing and, ultimately, time. Drug development is simply a time-consuming process—and the reason it takes time is because it can be a dangerous game to make big claims before the research backs those claims up and before a product has been adequately tested for safety and efficacy. Set against this backdrop, it becomes all the more obvious that the cannabis market as it stands now is making proclamations that science simply hasn't backed up.

Let me be clear: of all of the cannabis products on the market, *none* have gone through all of the steps mentioned in the previous section. No product has been backed by the rigors of the research process that other medicines must undergo. It pains me that we have left the cannabis industry to those who have no scientific or medical background to be making the ostentatious claims you hear today. But they seem to be the largest group of people conscious of the capabilities of the plant. Without their voice, who is going to wake my colleagues up? The medical cannabis market offers a lot of hype—but the plant itself is undeniably healing and potentially miraculous. Instead of overhyping or overdramatizing either positive or negative claims, we should be focusing our efforts on determining its dynamicity and unlocked potential, with patience and care.

But in the meantime, what are some of these claims we're referring to—and why are they so off base? Let's take a look.

CANNABIS CLAIMS, DEMYSTIFIED

By the time I was searching for a CBD product for Macario, I had been in the world of science for nearly a decade—I knew the aforementioned protocols well. I wasn't expecting a medicinal-grade product, but I did expect more consistency. What I was hoping for was a truly pure oil containing cannabidiol—that is, an oil with that single molecular compound, repeated over and over. My time as a biologist underscored the need for purity. We spend decades studying a single compound under our microscopes, because once you add one compound to another, entirely new reactions can occur.

The claims of cannabidiol were enough for this mother to give it a chance. But every CBD oil I tested had filler products that I knew could change the compound and make it less potent or reactive in other unknown ways. The variability not only between products but, more strikingly, between different vials of the same product was completely unexpected. Given what I wanted to do for Macario—wean him off his medications entirely—I simply couldn't administer anything with fillers or other cannabinoids that I did not know enough about to determine what they might do once inside my son's bloodstream. For anyone seeking to use cannabis as medicine, they'd do well to consider the same for themselves.

The process of making medicine has its flaws, but one guarantee we can always find with medicine is that we know what's in it. Like anything else, when we don't know what's in the products we ingest, we're dealing with a certain amount of risk—and we are not guaranteed results can be replicated even in our own bodies from product to product.

I went cold turkey on all of Macario's pharmaceutical medications. I would not feel confident in recommending the same regimen

I administered Macario to any other parent—even if their child's condition matched Macario's exactly, from the epileptic battle to the brain resection. The reason for this is twofold: first, no child would have the exact issue as Macario, because every child is genetically different from one another, and those dissimilarities must be treated on a case-by-case basis. But more importantly, the mechanism behind my CBD oil helping Macario still has not been fully explained—and it would take at least a decade to do so. As a scientist, it would simply be irresponsible to prescribe anything that we cannot understand. While it may work, it also might not—and then what?

It is because of both my professional and personal experience that I am cautious about cannabis claims, including the claims I can make based on my own son's recovery. In the next sections, I outline just a few of the most popular pro- and anticannabis claims, with the goal of providing clarity about why caution might just be the only way of moving forward in the industry writ large.

PRO-CANNABIS CLAIM: THE ENTOURAGE EFFECT

If you were to visit a reputable cannabis dispensary in any of the states or countries where the plant is legal to consume, you'd likely see signs listing the ratios of various cannabinoids in each strain and providing detailed information about terpenes and flavonoids. For newbies to the cannabis industry, those details can read quite confusingly—"Don't I just need something with THC or CBD?" they might ask. The dispensary staff would nod knowingly and then explain one of the most popularly held theories in cannabis culture today: the entourage effect. This theory suggests that the many compounds within the cannabis plant—including THC, CBD, other cannabinoids, terpenes, and flavonoids—work together in a sort of synergy to bring about different impacts on your body and mind. Further, many proponents of this theory believe that because of this effect, botanical cannabis is more effective than isolated molecules from the plant, whether CBD or THC.

First coined in 1998 by Israeli scientists Raphael Mechoulam and Shimon Ben-Shabat, the entourage effect originally described a phenomenon within the body's endocannabinoid system in which a variety of inactive molecules within the cannabis plant produced enhanced activity of the primary endogenous cannabinoids.[53] Now, the entourage effect is more commonly used as a vocabulary term with a strong belief that the plant components will work together to provide more of a benefit to the endocannabinoid system. This may not be untrue, but it is certainly jumping the gun, because the few cannabinoids we know about can work so differently and even more so together. Until we've been able to define this synergy, it's a hypothesis that should not be an established treatment—at least not yet.

There's only one problem: all evidence for or against an entourage effect, whether from the dispensaries listing ratios on their signs or from scientists like me who look skeptically upon such a theory, is purely anecdotal. Botanical cannabis has not been thoroughly shown to be more effective than its isolated counterparts. If so, the research is hard to trust because of the variability that would come with the botanical control or extract products. Certain strains have not been proven to make you sleepy or awake. Every person is different. And now that the entourage effect has been co-opted as another marketing term for dispensaries to use to lend legitimacy to their product, it's become all the more difficult to remind consumers that what may

---

53   Ethan B. Russo, "The case for the entourage effect and conventional breeding of clinical cannabis," *Frontiers in Plant Science*, January 9, 2019, https://www.ncbi.nlm.nih.gov/pmc/articles/PMC6334252/.

really be contributing to their specific highs is a placebo effect rather than anything innate in a bud of cannabis itself.[54]

Our ability to digest and metabolize substances is a critical element of our health, and it's entirely possible that something like an entourage effect is real. But until we truly meet this claim with the scientific rigor it deserves, we aren't doing due diligence to the potential of the plant. If such an effect does exist, we'd do well to understand it so that we could create more defined entourage effects that work in expected manners for patients. And if it does not work, we can have a next clear-cut cannabinoid product for them to try. Because again, every person is different. And if it doesn't exist, we'd still do well in understanding how the various cannabinoids, terpenes, and flavonoids are being metabolized in the body so we know exactly why we wouldn't want them in a medicine-grade substance. I don't have an issue with plants being marketed for the highs they give consumers— but I do have a problem with those plants being marketed for the therapeutic benefits they offer. Those claims need to be backed by research—and right now, they are not.

PRO-CANNABIS CLAIM: CBD COUNTERACTS THC

A claim arising from the entourage effect is the increasingly pervasive idea that the nonpsychoactive properties of CBD can work synergistically to balance out, mitigate, or even counteract the psychoactive properties of THC. Tetrahydrocannabinol is the primary psychoactive compound in the cannabis plant, and while it has been shown to

---

54   Angus Chen, "Some of the parts: Is marijuana's entourage effect scientifically valid?," *Scientific American*, April 20, 2017, https://www.scientificamerican.com/article/some-of-the-parts-is-marijuana-rsquo-s-ldquo-entourage-effect-rdquo-scientifi-cally-valid/.

relieve symptoms like pain and nausea, it can also cause side effects that many would rather avoid, including dizziness, paranoia, anxiety, and more. In general, the claims suggest CBD can impact the negative symptoms by altering the way THC binds to the body's endocannabinoid receptors. However, those claims have been across the board when it comes to simple administration, with some reports suggesting CBD should be taken before THC in order to reduce the symptoms and others suggesting they need to be taken together. None of the claims have been backed up by solid scientific research.[55]

Again—perhaps CBD does indeed have a mitigating effect or synergistic relationship with THC. But when it came to the administration of a product for my son, there was no way I could rely on "perhaps" as an answer. If we want to bring legitimacy into the world of cannabis, we need to take a step back, study each cannabinoid in isolation, as well as each terpene and flavonoid, and get a better sense of what we're working with. We need to bring our amazing technological advancements into the cannabis space and really define the botanicals at work. If there's synergy—great. If there's not—that's great, too, because then we'll know. But without knowing, we don't have a chance to fight to change this industry.

PRO-CANNABIS CLAIM: THC KILLS CANCER CELLS

Every cannabis claim not backed up by the research tends to overgeneralize both the compounds within the plant itself and the problem it supposedly targets. The entourage effect, for instance, claims "x:y:z ratio aids sleep"—but what do we really know about the x, y, and z

---

55   Raymond J.M. Niesink et al., "Does cannabidiol protect against adverse psychological effects of THC?," *Frontiers in Psychiatry*, April 2013: 130, https://www.ncbi.nlm.nih.gov/pmc/articles/PMC3797438/.

molecules in the ratio? What do we even know about them alone? And what do we know about sleep? We need science to answer the former, but for the latter, we know there are multiple factors contributing to rest and wakefulness. Could a plant target sleep wholesale and guarantee a good rest for all who buy that strain?

It's certainly a bold claim—but I know a claim that's bolder: that cannabis cures cancer. According to one recent analysis, in 2019 "the use of cannabis as a cancer cure represented the largest category (23.5%) of social media content on alternative cancer treatments. The top false news story claiming cannabis as a cancer cure generated 4.26 million engagements on social media, while the top accurate news story debunking this false news generated .0036 million engagements."[56]

This is the type of hype that is particularly worrisome to me. My own family and I sought out alternative cancer treatments for my father—and we are very much a part of a growing movement of individuals doing so. But when an article or "news" is published that capitalizes on this movement for the benefit of some cannabis marketer's greedy pockets, I get frustrated. Not only do we not understand the full benefits of THC, let alone the rest of the plant, but to say any single substance cures cancer is to greatly diminish the complexity of the disease itself. Every single type of cancer cell is different—and it's dangerous to suggest before rigorous research that one substance could cure them all.

To take it one step further, if there were a cannabis substance to cure cancer, it wouldn't be found on the shelves of any current dispensary. It would be the product of years of drug development— otherwise, there would never be a guarantee of replicability across populations. It's endlessly worrisome to see cannabis being peddled

---

56   Siyu Shi et al., "False news of a cannabis cancer cure," *Cureus*, January 2019; 11(1): e3918, https://www.ncbi.nlm.nih.gov/pmc/articles/PMC6426557/.

by sellers as some sort of cure-all when what's really on the shelves right now is not medicine. It's entertainment. We must start underscoring the difference.

What's really on the shelves right now is not medicine. It's entertainment.

ANTICANNABIS CLAIM: CBD CAUSES LIVER DAMAGE

Pro-cannabis claims, of course, are just one part of the story. Balancing out the onslaught of dubious good news from the entertainment cannabis industry is a litter of rumors warning of specific dangers from the plant that are just as unproven by the research. Unfortunately, some of those negative claims have come from entities that should know better than to make a claim before the research has proven it definitively one way or the other.

In the spring of 2019, a study was published in the scientific magazine *Molecules* that suggested cannabidiol could lead to liver damage. As the abstract states, "CBD exhibited clear signs of hepatotoxicity" and "raises serious concerns about potential drug interactions as well as the safety of CBD."[57] The researchers concluded by underscoring the need for more research above all in order to evaluate CBD's safety and potential long-term health risks. They also noted the object of their particular study was Epidiolex, the first FDA-approved cannabidiol prescription medication on the market, and that the study of other CBD products as they come to market may not lead to the same findings.[58]

---

57   Laura Ewing et al., "Hepatotoxicity of a cannabidiol-rich cannabis extract in the mouse model," *Molecules*, 2019; 24(9): 1694, https://www.mdpi.com/1420-3049/24/9/1694.

58   Mike Adams, "Marijuana study finds CBD can cause liver damage," *Forbes*, last updated June 18, 2019, https://www.forbes.com/sites/mikeadams/2019/06/18/marijuana-study-finds-cbd-can-cause-liver-damage/#1b2ef0a243ff.

The FDA has noted this claim several times in its press releases and other literature about CBD products and testing, with one recent release stating the potential for liver injury represents a serious risk that "can be managed when the product is taken under medical supervision in accordance with the FDA-approved labeling for the product, but it is less clear how this risk might be managed in a setting where this drug substance is used far more widely, without medical supervision and not in accordance with FDA-approved labeling." The release continues, "There are also unresolved questions regarding the cumulative exposure to CBD if people access it across a broad range of consumer products as well as questions regarding the intended functionality of CBD in such products. Additionally, there are open questions about whether some threshold level of CBD could be allowed in foods without undermining the drug approval process or diminishing commercial incentives for further clinical study of the relevant drug substance."[59]

The release continues with a call for comments, data, and information about CBD, including what levels of cannabis cause safety concerns, how the various modes of delivery may affect the safety of these compounds, and how cannabis and cannabis-derived compounds interact with other substances.

The release's call for information to be submitted for review belies the agency's seeming quickness to jump on the claim that CBD causes liver damage. Without that additional information, can we really claim this at all? We need far more studies to be done on exactly the topics the FDA is calling for—dosage, mode of delivery, and other interactions—before we can safely assume toxicity to be a problem with CBD medicines. To propagate this claim is to enter into the same

---

59   "FDA Statement," FDA, last updated April 2, 2019, https://www.fda.gov/news-events/press-announcements/statement-fda-commissioner-scott-gottlieb-md-new-steps-advance-agencys-continued-evaluation.

problem as those who seek to spread positive information about the plant. Both are under-researched and overstated.

ANTICANNABIS CLAIM: VAPING CAUSES LUNG DISEASE

In fall of 2019, stories of the dangers of vaping hit a critical mass. In September 2019, the CEO of Juul, the most widely known vape company, stepped down amid controversies that the company courted younger users and misrepresented its product as less harmful than smoking. Over five hundred cases of lung illnesses tied to vaping were reported, as well as at least nine deaths,[60] with both numbers inevitably set to rise in the coming months. Several of those illnesses were tied to vaping cannabis oil—leading many to suggest vaping marijuana can be significantly detrimental to health.[61]

Ultimately, this comes down to a regulation issue and a research issue. Vapes exploded onto the market in relative recency, and there's been decades more research on their cigarette counterparts than on vapes themselves. E-cigarettes, or vapes, work by heating substances—most commonly liquid nicotine or cannabis oil—into aerosols that can then be inhaled. On its face, it seems this method of inhalation would be healthier than cigarettes, which use simple combustion as its method of inhalation—leading to nasty by-products like tar and chemicals to be inhaled along with the substances itself. But there's just not enough evidence in the vape market to back up any signifi-

60   Jim Zarroli, "Juul's CEO steps down amid controversy over vaping," NPR, September 25, 2019, https://www.npr.org/2019/09/25/764390058/juuls-ceo-steps-down-amid-controversy-over-vaping.

61   Jayne O'Donnell et al., "People are vaping THC. Lung injuries reported nationwide. Why is the CDC staying quiet?," USA Today, August 28, 2019, https://www.usatoday.com/story/news/health/2019/08/28/critics-cdc-silent-vaping-thc-injuries-mount/2121523001/.

cant claims. There's not enough evidence to suggest vaping cannabis products causes lung damage, and there's not enough evidence to suggest vaping itself was ever a healthier alternative.

The public health crisis we have on our hands now with vaping is entirely due to a product with extraordinary claims coming to market before any of those claims could really be researched. We are now at risk of doing the same thing with cannabis products writ large—and the act of putting the cart before the horse must stop.

ANTICANNABIS CLAIM: THC CAUSES SCHIZOPHRENIA

The idea that heavy cannabis use could lead to psychosis was first conceived almost a century ago, when the movie *Reefer Madness* invoked a mass cultural hysteria about marijuana use leading to dire consequences, from murderous rampages to flat-out insanity. A church group initially funded and made the film as a sort of moral fable to show children the dangers of cannabis. But the film quickly took on a life of its own, catching fire across the country and sparking fear in the hearts of many.

The film undoubtedly played a role in changing public opinion about cannabis—just a year after the film's initial release in 1936, congress passed the Marijuana Tax Act, effectively criminalizing the plant across the country. This law laid the groundwork for the restrictions scientists continue to face today as they seek to study the medicinal benefits of cannabis.[62]

Perhaps you can therefore understand how much it pains me to hear rumors linking cannabis to mental illness reinserting themselves

---

62   Matthew Green, "Reefer madness! The twisted history of America's weed laws," KQED, January 5, 2018, https://www.kqed.org/lowdown/24153/reefer-madness-the-twisted-history-of-americas-weed-laws.

into the cultural fabric. The fact is, any number of substances can cause an adverse reaction in our bodies if we ingest too much of them. We can drink too much caffeine; we can drink too much alcohol. But there is absolutely no evidence whatsoever of a connection between schizophrenia and THC use.

Some who oppose this perspective cite the fact that numerous studies have shown a correlation between regular cannabis use and psychotic problems arising for the user—but this remains a hotly contested debate among people within the industry, who underscore that correlation does not necessarily equal causation. Once again, this claim goes far beyond the research and overgeneralizes cannabis itself and the origins of mental illness, which can arise from a multiplicity of factors, including inherited risk.[63]

* * *

The move to legalize cannabis use in the United States is overwhelmingly positive and a step in the right direction in moving past the decades-old stereotypes that the plant has never quite been able to shake. However, legalizing cannabis and utilizing the plant in drug development for the eventual purpose of medicinal use are two very different things—and our research in the latter remains limited at best. Legalization has not yet made its way to the research labs, where cannabis's status as a Schedule 1 controlled substance limits potential for studies to back up or disprove the countless dubious claims, both positive and negative, about the plant. And given the fact most drug development timelines average a decade and a half at minimum, it's concerning to think what other claims may arise

---

63   Benedict Carey, "Does marijuana use cause schizophrenia?," *The New York Times*, January 17, 2019, https://www.nytimes.com/2019/01/17/health/cannabis-marijuana-schizophrenia.html.

between our current era and a future era where studies may theoretically become easier to conduct.

We all know the field needs more research—and it is my hope that this chapter has shed light on what that really means and why it's so important. The future of cannabis is already here, whether we like it or not—will we as a culture continue to let the disinformation about this plant spread, while its true potential gets lost in the shuffle of time?

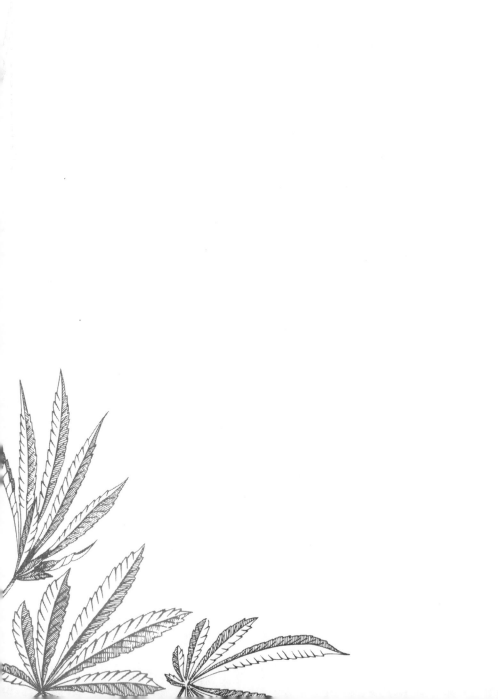

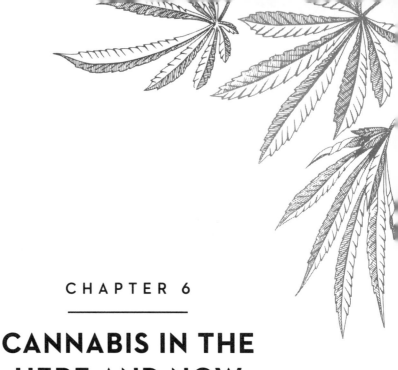

CHAPTER 6

CANNABIS IN THE HERE AND NOW

After the pure CBD oil I developed for my son led to his remarkable recovery, I knew I had made a medicine that could have the power to change lives—and possibly change the world. CBD had given my son a chance at a future. While acknowledging the lack of rigorous research and medical standards around the cannabis industry, I knew what kind of product I had made, and began to wonder how far its impact could go.

As the months passed, I began to see how embedded the misinformation on the current cannabis market is in our culture. Stereotypes about the plant run rampant and lead people to develop opinions, both positive and negative, based on hype alone. As I saw the market for CBD products explode, with CBD-infused coffee, ice cream, candies, and more being sold everywhere from the pharmacy to the video store, I saw a shift happen among my friends and acquaintances. Cannabidiol, the same compound that saved my son, from the same plant with thousands of years of healing traditions behind it across the globe, was now becoming a contemporary snake oil, something to be looked upon with the utmost skepticism rather than the utmost curiosity.

Several months after I developed the CBD oil that changed Macario's life, I went for coffee with a friend who is one of the biggest nonbelievers in the cannabis hype spreading through our cultural consciousness. He works out frequently, and as we chatted, he started asking questions about whether the CBD oil I developed could help with his pain and recovery. I took out a bottle of my CBD oil and offered him a dropperful. A few minutes passed, and my friend grew quiet, but his facial expressions and movements suggested something was going on in his body that his mind was trying to process. A few more minutes later, he spoke. He had been struggling with acid reflux for the better part of seven years. Within minutes of taking the CBD oil, his acid reflux was gone—and it stayed gone.

Similarly, I administered the CBD oil to a woman with dystonia, who had significant muscle spasms in her face that kept her from carrying on a regular conversation and made her feel frequently embarrassed. After consistently taking the CBD for three months, she sent me a text telling me she'd had a few of the best days of her life.

In the last chapter, I underscored the point that anecdotal evidence is not enough, and that claims beyond the research don't serve the cannabis industry and may in fact harm the long-term reputation of the plant's healing capacities. For me, the transformations I've seen with my own eyes do not equate to good science, but they do have a valuable message for me—and all of us—about cannabis: we may not yet have the hows and whys about what's happening, but something is, indeed, happening, when suffering patients ingest cannabis. And that brings us to the central theme of this chapter: what is going on with the state of the industry right now? What do we know, what don't we know, and what should we be aware of as we move forward?

The mounting anecdotal evidence I've accumulated, including the stories just mentioned of friends who have found relief by using CBD, aptly highlight each of the three core elements of the state of today's cannabis industry that I'll explore in depth in the pages that follow:

> We may not yet have the hows and whys about what's happening, but something is, indeed, happening, when suffering patients ingest cannabis.

- First, how are we to measure whether cannabis and more specifically cannabidiol have truly healing properties within the molecules, or whether the anecdotal impacts are a simple indicator of a placebo effect at work?

- Second, what specific complexities stand in the way of anecdotal evidence being enough for now, as the industry catches up?

- Third, what are we to make of the multiple means of administering cannabis on the market right now?

- How do each of these three factors interact and influence one another?

This broad overview of trends in the CBD and cannabis space is meant to provide a solid foundation from which we can launch as we turn to the last chapter of the book: the future.

WHAT IS THE PLACEBO EFFECT— AND WHY DOES IT MATTER?

Thanks to the twenty-first century's implicit prioritization of hyper-productivity, efficiency, optimization, and always-on-ness, we are collectively always on the lookout for an easy fix to our overwhelm. Since the early aughts, rotating lists of superfoods have risen to the challenge, with varying degrees of success. One superfood that continues to hold the spotlight in health-food circles is coconut oil. The claims were perfectly tailored to the needs of a stressed-out populace with too much to do and too little time: coconut oil "blasted" belly fat, bolstered the immune system, staved off cognitive decline, and curbed the appetite.[64] The oil remains popular among those practicing a ketogenic or paleo-based diet. Much like the anecdotal evidence we see in the cannabis industry, coconut oil had numerous proponents, ranging from the celebrity to the local holistic practitioner. And just as with cannabis, skeptics began to wonder: how much of the efficacy of the oil (if any!) was due to the oil itself—and how much could be attributed to the placebo effect?

THE PLACEBO EFFECT, EXPLAINED

Introduced in the late eighteenth century, the term *placebo* was used to describe the prescription of an inert substance—like a sugar pill or a mild ointment—to "satisfy the patient's demand and his expectations," or, more specifically, to satisfy his or her obstinate mind.[65] Because of the questionable ethics involved in prescribing a placebo in the place of a drug of substance, placebo is often used in pop culture

---

64   "The nutrition source," Harvard University, accessed April 2020, https://www.hsph.harvard.edu/nutritionsource/food-features/coconut-oil/.

65   Robert Jütte, "The early history of the placebo," *Complementary Therapies in Medicine*, April 2013; 21(2): 94–7, https://www.ncbi.nlm.nih.gov/pubmed/23497809.

as a dirty word or an ineffective treatment—when in fact, this could not be further from the truth.

Thus far in the book, I have frequently discussed the holistic, unpredictable forces at play that can make or break a health outcome. My father was not supposed to survive his cancer diagnosis. Macario was not supposed to be developing as he is today, a normal, regular kid. The placebo effect underscores how incredible the mind can be as a tool to heal the body, and how much we have yet to learn about the interconnectedness of our bodies, minds, and environments.

A placebo may be an inert medication, but researchers have found the placebo effect can be just as effective as the real thing for certain conditions. Their studies show that when a patient undergoes the ritual of treatment—which includes everything from making the appointment to sitting in the medical facility's waiting room to being examined by a doctor and eventually picking up a bottle of pills at a pharmacy and swallowing a pill with the confidence it will help ease symptoms—the patient's brain releases a healthy dose of feel-good neurotransmitters linked to better mood and lower stress.[66] That release can significantly shift a patient's subjective experience of their symptoms. A placebo may not cure cancer—it cannot shrink a tumor or lower bad cholesterol—but it can lessen pain, reduce fatigue, and ease nausea.

Ted Kaptchuk, the Director of Harvard University's Program in Placebo Studies and the Therapeutic Encounter, and a leading researcher on the placebo effect, suggests the efficacy of the placebo demonstrates that basic compassion and trust in a care provider have real impact in a patient's health outcomes—and that low-tech placebos have something valuable to contribute to high-tech proce-

---

66   "The power of the placebo effect," Harvard University, last updated August 9, 2019, https://www.health.harvard.edu/mental-health/the-power-of-the-placebo-effect.

dures.[67] Given the strength of the placebo, it makes sense that the gold standard of medications entering the market is to prove themselves stronger than the sugar pill—after all, if an inert substance could treat you just as well as a prescription med, why the need for the medicine in the first place?

THE DOUBLE-BLIND STUDY

In chapters 4 and 5, I introduced you to the rigorous process of testing that every medicine must undergo before making it to market. One of the most important tests of all—the make-or-break test for any pill—is what's known as a double-blind, placebo-controlled study. In these studies, half of the participant pool receives a real medication and the other half receives a placebo, designed to appear as much like the real thing as possible. The participants do not know which pill they're taking—in other words, they're blind. The study is double blind because the participants aren't the only ones in the dark about which pill is which in treatment. The researchers administering the two pills also do not know which is which; this reduces any possible unintentional bias or tip-off that could alter the results of the study.[68] If the placebo performs as well or better than the medication, the medication is clearly not of use. If the medication performs significantly better, this study is a strong indication that the medication does indeed have something of value to offer in terms of treatment.

---

67   "One scholar's take on the power of the placebo," NPR, last updated January 6, 2012, https://www.npr.org/2012/01/06/144794035/one-scholars-take-on-the-power-of-the-placebo.

68   Shobha Misra, "Randomized double blind placebo control studies, the 'Gold Standard' in intervention based studies," *Indian Journal of Sexually Transmitted Diseases and AIDS*, July-December 2012; 33(2): 131–134, https://www.ncbi.nlm.nih.gov/pmc/articles/PMC3505292/.

WHY DOES THE PLACEBO MATTER
IN CANNABIS RESEARCH?

The mind is a powerful thing—and the power of our own beliefs can have a strong influence on certain health outcomes. But placebo alone is not good enough. Outside of the lab, the placebo effect of certain superfoods or other remedies should not detract us from investigating whether those superfoods or remedies could perform with even greater efficacy. It should not detract us, in other words, from continuing to distill our knowledge of a treatment down to the molecular level to determine whether the mechanism of action truly is a placebo—in other words, whether the superfood is just a more expensive sugar pill—or if there's a real biological reaction taking place to produce change.

Let's return to the example of coconut oil. With so many brands of coconut oil on the market and different methods of production, what, exactly, if anything, was at the root of the claims that this oil could be the next weight-loss miracle? The answer could be found under the microscope and in the lab. Coconut oil contains a mix of two different types of fats: medium-chain triglycerides (MCTs) and long-chain triglycerides (LCTs). Studies show that MCTs are processed different than their long-chain counterparts in ways that can both satiate the appetite and lead to greater fat loss.[69] The distillation of a holistic product into its most effective compound has allowed for the creation of a more specific product that has a greater impact. Removed from the other fillers found in regular coconut oil, MCT oil is a far more potent weight-loss product than its alternative—and far more promising.

---

69   Marie-Pierre St-Onge et al., "Weight-loss diet that includes consumption of medium-chain triacylglycerol oil leads to a greater rate of weight and fat mass loss than does olive oil," *The American Journal of Clinical Nutrition*, March 2008; 87(3): 621–626, https://www.ncbi.nlm.nih.gov/pmc/articles/PMC2874190/.

Cannabis is like coconut oil—and cannabidiol is its MCT. However, THC and CBD are just two of the many potential compounds within the cannabis plant, and as with coconut oil, it's impossible to know which are just fillers and which are effective remedies with significant treatment potential without looking under the microscope and conducting studies. As discussed in chapter 5, the entourage effect, or the idea that all chemical compounds within CBD need each other and work together to create a given medicinal outcome, has not been proven. The only evidence we have of every molecule working together in a beneficial way is the growth of the plant itself. Until we isolate the cannabinoids one by one, and the terpenes one by one, and understand whether and how they are beneficial by themselves, we cannot possibly understand how they are beneficial together.

When people take a pill they believe will have an impact on their health, they're engaging in the chain reaction of the placebo effect—and they may see some beneficial health outcomes. Likewise, when you take a sip of a CBD latte and believe it will lower your anxiety, you may find your anxiety indeed lessen over the course of the day. But given the unrefined nature of the products on the market, the lack of regulation or oversight as to what and how much is in a product, and the fillers that may be masking or lessening the potency of the CBD itself, it's safe to assume if your anxiety goes down, it's probably not the CBD. It is probably the placebo effect.

The placebo is not a good enough standard for cannabis as a medicine—and we should expect more from our products today and in the future. Only research will get us there. If your goal is to lose weight, why take coconut oil if you can take MCT? We need to ask ourselves similar questions about cannabis, CBD, and the desired outcomes we may come to expect in the future from the many cannabinoids and other molecules found in the cannabis leaf.

DOSING DIFFICULTIES

Here are a few jarring insights into today's cannabis market. In part because the legal market is so young, there are no universal standards when it comes to testing and labeling of products. Despite the fact that many states require such standards, a recent study published in the *Journal of the American Medical Association* found that, of seventy-five products obtained and tested from markets in Los Angeles, San Francisco, and Seattle, just 17 percent were labeled accurately.[70] Another recent study, published in the *Annals of Internal Medicine*, determined that cannabis-related visits to the emergency room have tripled in Colorado since the drug became legal for recreation in 2014.[71] Since 1995, THC levels found in cannabis have nearly tripled[72]—and medical practitioners have such little clarity in terms of whether and how to prescribe cannabis in the first place that figuring out proper dosing seems like two or three steps further down the road.

> Medical practitioners have such little clarity in terms of whether and how to prescribe cannabis in the first place that figuring out proper dosing seems like two or three steps further down the road.

70   Ryan Vandrey et al., "Cannabinoid dose and label accuracy in edible medical cannabis products," *JAMA*, 2015, 313(24): 2491–2493, https://jamanetwork.com/journals/jama/fullarticle/2338239.

71   Andrew A. Monte et al., "Acute illness associated with cannabis use, by route of exposure: an observational study," *Annals of Internal Medicine*, April 16, 2019, https://annals.org/aim/article-abstract/2729208/acute-illness-associated-cannabis-use-route-exposure-observational-study.

72   Matt Simon, "Why it's so hard to dose weed," *WIRED*, last updated February 26, 2018, https://www.wired.com/story/why-its-so-hard-to-dose-weed/.

It's a point that I've reiterated several times throughout this book, but is worth underscoring yet again: as long as cannabis remains a Schedule 1 drug under the Federal Controlled Substances Act—meaning the federal government believes there is no accepted medical use for this plant and a high potential for abuse—cannabis research will be severely constrained. And if the research is limited by the law, there can be no expectation of scientifically backed standards for testing products and labeling their ingredients. There can also be no expectation of dosing standards. And without that scientific rigor, how can we expect cannabis companies to be able to understand the molecular intricacies of their own product, let alone explain to consumers what's in it and why?

In a country like Canada, my birthplace, where cannabis is federally legal, the research potential is extensive when juxtaposed against the barriers the US places on the very same studies. However, from what I've seen thus far, the legalization of marijuana in Canada has had more of a recreational and financial benefit than a medical benefit. Worldwide, the problems are the same. There is no true understanding or guidance on what type of products to make per specific condition, how to dose, and what the expected outcomes may be. And rightfully so: this plant is complex and will take many great minds and a lot of time—we're only just beginning, but the market should recognize where we are and not pretend we're somewhere further along.

All of this has created the perfect storm for current cannabis dosing trends. Simply put, they're something of a disaster. Proper cannabis dosing depends on a variety of factors, from delivery method (for instance, is a patient ingesting cannabis via inhalation or sublingually?) to prior usage of the drug (has the patient developed a tolerance?). A dose that works for one person could land another in the emergency room. It's not the plant's fault—it's simply the fact that we don't have enough information at our fingertips to understand which molecules from the plant are doing what, and how much of each molecule is needed for effective treatment.[73]

With prescription medicine, dosing is possible because the molecular makeup of each pill is exactly the same. Not all CBD oils are created equally—and undoubtedly, no two joints, tinctures, or other administrations of cannabis look alike. But there's another problem embedded in the classification of cannabis as a Schedule 1 drug. Not only does the label limit researchers from investigating the plant but it also limits a doctor's ability to prescribe cannabis as a medicine at all.

As I discussed in chapter 4, the Upstairs Downstairs effect inhibits clear and frequent communication between researchers and medical practitioners. But as is the case with cannabis, there can be no communication if there is no research to begin with. Ethical questions may arise for doctors who seek to prescribe cannabis freely available on the market—and that means patients are essentially left to their own devices if they want to give medical marijuana a try. In writing an opinion piece for *STAT*, a journal covering the latest developments in the life sciences and academic labs, one individual put it best:

---

73   Kevin Joy, "Legalized cannabis brings new challenges for health care providers," Michigan Medicine, last updated June 4, 2019, https://labblog.uofmhealth.org/industry-dx/marijuana-intoxication-at-emergency-departments-perfcon.

"Until there's some real change [in the medical cannabis industry], like making it easier to study the effects of medical marijuana and also training doctors about its benefits and risks, we will all continue to be dazed and confused."[74]

Dosing concerns are a matter I hold close to my heart. The first published research on dosing on children using CBD for epilepsy suggested patients ingest 5 mg/kg of body weight. That's like drinking several tincture bottles of the 3,000 mg FDA-approved CBD we currently have on the market per day. Therapeutically, thousands of milligrams of CBD were needed to penetrate the cells to have an effect. Our bodies can only absorb so much of any given substance. Meanwhile, the motto for THC dosing has historically been: go slow and titrate up based on your tolerance. How much longer can this last? Researchers seem to agree on one thing: "With the advent of pharmaceutical cannabis-based medicines (Sativex and Epidiolex) and liberalization of access in certain nations, this ignorance of cannabis pharmacology and therapeutics has become untenable."[75]

> Until we open up pathways to research, dosing will remain a significant concern for today's cannabis market.

Until we open up pathways to research, dosing will remain a significant concern for today's cannabis market. But as previously mentioned, method of administration plays a key role in determining

---

74   Shari Berman, "I wanted to try medical marijuana. Why couldn't my doctors help me?," *STAT*, last updated July 19, 2019, https://www.statnews.com/2019/07/19/medical-marijuana-doctors-no-help/.

75   Caroline A. MacCallum et al., "Practical considerations in medical cannabis administration and dosing," *European Journal of Internal Medicine*, January 4, 2018, https://www.ejinme.com/article/S0953-6205(18)30004-9/pdf.

how much cannabis should be ingested. With that in mind, let's take a broad look at the methods on the market today, what each method can offer, and which challenges each method may pose to patients turning to cannabis as a therapeutic remedy for their ailments.

METHODS OF ADMINISTRATION

As I began my journey in the cannabis space, spreading the word about the amazing plant that saved my son, I realized early on that the cannabis market is significantly lacking in scientific expertise on the products they are trying to sell. As previously mentioned, the continued taboo of the plant keeps many researchers and doctors away, fearing their reputations might be smudged by being aligned with cannabis—a substance so maligned in recent history. What happened with Macario was too important for me to keep quiet about—and because I was not afraid to stake my professional reputation on the potential this plant has to heal the world, I fielded a lot of questions from eager consumers who had no one else to turn to for answers. Some of those questions were strikingly similar.

Many individuals asked how much cannabis they should take to see a result—and for reasons described in the prior section, I had no simple answer to give them. But many others asked questions about whether vaping was bad for them, if a topical ointment was as good as a tincture, and much more. These questions also did not lend themselves to a simple answer—perhaps someday they will, but not yet.

> My interest is in telling the truth in order to make change.

The truth of the matter is, I'm not interested in being opinionated about what method of administration works best and why. Rather, my interest is in telling the truth in order to make change. Over the course of my research and advocacy in the cannabis space, I've often wondered if individuals place too much of their opinions in the answers they give. I've also wondered at the power of good marketing to promote one method over the other. CBD oil is having a pop cultural moment right now—and yet, for the same reasons coconut oil and MCT are different from one another, CBD oil is not necessarily any better or worse in terms of administration than any other method. Most CBD oils on the market contain not just cannabidiol but also terpenes, flavonoids, chlorophyll, and many other substances that could very well be reactant—and the same goes for most other products on the market today.

With that in mind, my goal for this section is not to promote one method of administration over the other—at this point, you likely already know my claim: we need more research on all of them! Instead, I want to provide a broad overview of what's available right now on the market, to set the tone for what we might come to expect in the future.

THE FOUR METHODS

Currently, there are four methods of cannabis administration that nearly all products fall into: inhalation, oral administration, sublingual administration, and topical administration. Our body processes cannabinoids differently in each of these methods, and the chemical makeup of products within each category can further differentiate the effects of ingestion. Cannabis consumption is a complex matrix of administration and impact, and each of these has benefits and drawbacks, ranging from duration to concentration. In the future, it may make sense for professionals to work with specific symptoms described by patients and administer a product from one or multiple of these categories that is most optimal. Research and time will tell how these categories become more specified and precise—and I have high hopes that each will.

INHALATION

Inhalation of cannabis remains the most popular method of ingestion—and, because inhaled cannabinoids cross immediately the blood–brain barrier, it also offers the most immediate impact in terms of effects. Patients who smoke or vape cannabis feel its impact within minutes, with absorption levels peaking around one to two hours from initial inhalation.[76] Intoxication from inhalation can last anywhere from two to four hours.

Smoking and vaping share a commonality in their speedy delivery of molecules into our bloodstream, but there are important differences between these two methods of inhalation that can impact its effects. Smoking of the plant involves burning and inhaling dried cannabis flowers and adjacent leaves. The combustion of any material, whether cannabis, tobacco, or wood, releases toxins and carcinogens in the resulting smoke that can be harmful to lung health.[77] Burning cannabis can also lessen the amount of cannabinoids ingested versus the amount initially present in the flower and leaves, as some of the product is lost to exhalation, combustion, and other by-products of the smoke itself. Generally speaking, users absorb about 25 percent of cannabinoids present in cannabis when smoking the plant.[78] Of course, when taking into account the trend toward higher levels of THC found in the plant to begin with, this does not mean a joint is any less potent than any other means of ingestion.

---

76   Priyamvada Sharma et al., "Chemistry, Metabolism, and Toxicology of Cannabis: Clinical Implications," *Iranian Journal of Psychiatry*, Fall 2012; 7(4): 149–156, https://www.ncbi.nlm.nih.gov/pmc/articles/PMC3570572/.

77   "Marijuana and Lung Health," American Lung Association, accessed April 2020, https://www.lung.org/stop-smoking/smoking-facts/marijuana-and-lung-health.html.

78   Jeremy Peters et al., "Contemporary Routes of Cannabis Consumption: A Primer for Clinicians," *The Journal of the American Osteopathic Association*, February 2018; Volume 118, 67–70, https://jaoa.org/article.aspx?articleid=2671435.

Vaping was initially considered a healthier alternative to smoking because of the lack of side effects from the combustion and burning of the plant. Vaping typically involves inhaling cannabis that has been concentrated into an oil, which once heated can be inhaled as a vapor by the patient. While cannabis flowers can contain up to 20 percent THC, the oils used for vaping can contain significantly more—up to 80 percent.[79] Studies have also shown that patients absorb about 33 percent of cannabinoids found in the oil,[80] meaning that on nearly every metric, vaping offers a far more concentrated administration. As mentioned in the previous chapter, there have been some safety concerns around vaping, with a particular concern around the possible risk residues from the oil may pose to patient health. However, the answers we seek are not going to be found in speculation alone. As with everything in this industry, more testing is needed to determine tangible risks of this method of ingestion.[81]

Bottom line: Patients who are looking for an immediate impact on their symptoms, such as anxiety and pain, may look to inhalation as a useful method of administration.

ORAL ADMINISTRATION

Perhaps the next most popular method of cannabis ingestion is oral administration, in the form of edibles, capsules, oils, tinctures, and more. Unlike inhalation, in which patients can feel an immediate

---

79   "How marijuana is consumed," Drug Policy Alliance, accessed April 2020, http://www.drugpolicy.org/drug-facts/10-facts-about-marijuana/how-marijuana-consumed.

80   Jeremy Peters et al., "Contemporary Routes of Cannabis Consumption: A Primer for Clinicians," *The Journal of the American Osteopathic Association*, February 2018; Volume 118, 67–70, https://jaoa.org/article.aspx?articleid=2671435.

81   "How marijuana is consumed," Drug Policy Alliance, accessed April 2020, http://www.drugpolicy.org/drug-facts/10-facts-about-marijuana/how-marijuana-consumed.

effect of the cannabinoids entering their bloodstream, oral ingestion involves a longer process, with stronger results. Patients who consume cannabis feel its impact anywhere between thirty minutes to an hour. Like inhalation, absorption levels peak within about two hours, but the effects of the plant can linger for as long as six hours, and sometimes even more.

The impacts of oral ingestion differ significantly from inhalation because the cannabinoids are absorbed by the body using a different mechanism. Rather than immediately crossing the blood–brain barrier, as with inhalation, cannabinoids taken orally must first pass through the liver before reaching the brain. The liver then converts the cannabinoids into stronger and longer-lasting compounds. Because of the lack of immediacy and the passage through the liver, which can be highly variable in its absorption and conversion of substances (think of how alcohol is absorbed differently on an empty stomach, for instance, versus after a hearty meal), cannabis taken orally can pose a significant challenge when it comes to dosing. Still, oral ingestion may be a good option for patients who are looking for a longer-lasting relief to symptoms than inhalation may offer.

With any method of cannabis ingestion, there should be caution—especially with psychoactive cannabinoids. I've heard one too many stories of individuals, including my own husband, who loved the taste of a THC chocolate bar, ending up in a very shocked, nearly hallucinogenic, and uncomfortable state—one that lasts a lot longer than they expected.

SUBLINGUAL ADMINISTRATION

Sublingual administration of cannabis involves a patient applying drops of cannabis oil or a strip underneath their tongue and letting it dissolve. The sublingual cavity, or space beneath the tongue, is rich with blood vessels that can easily absorb cannabinoids. Thus, this method allows cannabis to be immediately absorbed into the bloodstream, with patients feeling their effects nearly as quickly as they would with inhalation. This method of administration is easier to dose and holds promise in the field of cannabis medicine—Sativex, the only FDA-approved cannabinoid medication on the market at the moment, is administered as a sublingual spray.

TOPICAL ADMINISTRATION

Lastly, cannabinoids can be absorbed through the skin using oils, lotions, salves, and even bath salts. However, our skin's complex system of absorption does not allow cannabinoids to enter into the bloodstream; instead, they interact with CB2 receptors close to our skin's surface without penetrating further. Because they do not enter the bloodstream, and thus do not have a pathway to the brain, topical cannabis treatments have the benefit of being nonpsychoactive, making them a good option for localized pain, like arthritis, cramping due to menstruation, and more.

There is one method of topical administration that does cross the blood–brain barrier, however. Cannabinoids found in transdermal patches can permeate through the protective layer of our skin and are absorbed slowly into the body over a period of time. While the effects of topical application usually last just one to two hours, transdermal patches can last for nearly two days.[82]

Whether our body is processing cannabinoids directly through the bloodstream or whether they're processed through the liver, we have all the right biological mechanisms to reap the benefits these potent chemicals may offer—both in terms of healing and in terms of relief. However, because we are not currently dealing with a market of regulated drugs that retain a modicum of consistency in terms of their outcomes, we must be wary of ingredients and by-products found in each of these categories that we may be unaware of or unaware of their consequences. There also needs to be greater transparency within the industry when it comes to potency and quality of the cannabis we are ingesting. Dosing is hard enough as it is in the market right now, but when products are not clearly and accurately labeled within each of these categories, patients are unable to clearly understand what may be working for them and why.

* * *

Here's what we know: Cannabis is a plant with a thousand-plus-year history of healing, grown and cultivated globally and widely accepted among a diversity of cultures—including in America—long before it became vilified and stigmatized in the twentieth century. Once vilified, the canon of knowledge we had about the plant was seemingly forgotten and the pathways forward in terms of future research stilted by restrictive laws. Now, with states legalizing cannabis, the plant is enjoying somewhat of a renaissance and its tainted status as a criminalized substance is beginning to wane in the popular culture. However, we are missing fundamental understandings about the plant that are preventing the current market from reaching its full potential.

---

82   Ibid, http://www.drugpolicy.org/drug-facts/10-facts-about-marijuana/how-marijuana-consumed.

Here is what we do not know: We do not know the full power of the cannabinoids we are currently most aware of—that is, CBD and THC—and how that power extends beyond the placebo. We do not know the potential power of the dozens of cannabinoids, terpenes, and other substances that make up the plant, and whether each should be filtered out for a stronger product or kept in for some synergistic benefit. We know that the placebo effect is powerful, but I believe cannabis strains are far stronger and objectively more healing. In the future, this should be the goal of any individual invested in understanding more about how the strong potential of cannabis ultimately pans out in the lab and eventually in the patient.

> We know that the placebo effect is powerful, but I believe cannabis strains are far stronger and objectively more healing.

Here is what we need to understand further: Dosing of cannabis must become an easier project to undertake—and in the future, it must not lie in the patient's own trial-and-error process to find out. Dosing threatens to undermine each of the four methods of cannabis administration I outlined in this chapter. If a patient ingests too much orally, they may be turned off from the plant for good. If the patient ingests too little sublingually, they may walk away from the treatment with the belief that there is little this plant has to offer them. Safety, too, threatens to undermine these methods. Vaping can easily be titrated and has an immediate impact, but if the oil being vaporized contains chemicals that otherwise hurt a patient's health, how can a doctor faithfully recommend this as a medication? Lastly, quality affects these methods. Topical ointments can only go so far if they're created with products that don't effectively absorb into the skin. Each of these presents a barrier to adequate dosing, to patient satisfaction, and to the industry itself.

Here is what I know: My son was saved via the administration of a powerful and potent CBD oil, directly administered through his feeding tube. My friend was cured of his acid reflux, and my other friend is on the road to being cured of her dystonia. Anecdotes will never be enough—but their tales of healing have the power to light the fire under an industry struggling to become legitimate and define itself against its reputation as entertainment, snake oil, or fad.

This may be what the industry offers now—but I'm confident we can move toward a brighter future. And I plan to do my part to get us there.

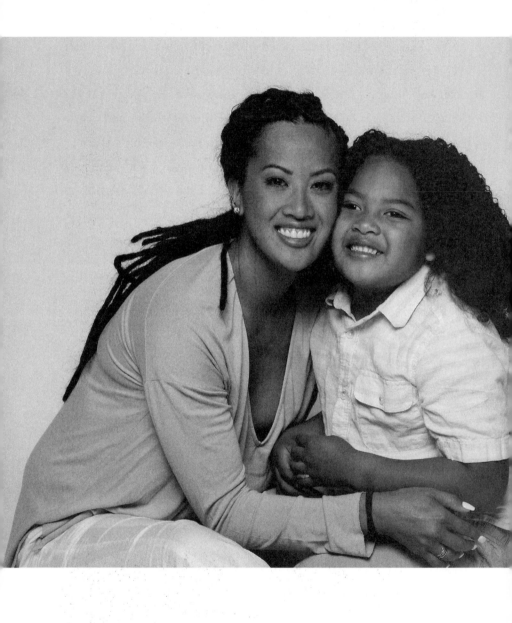

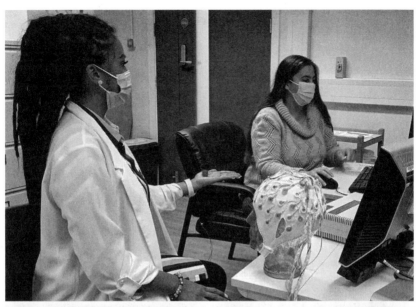

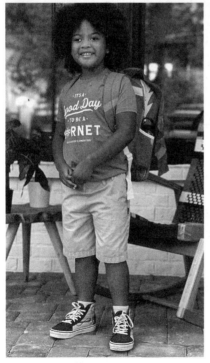

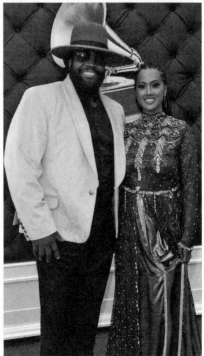

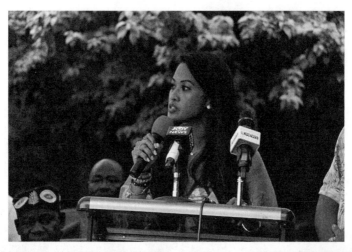

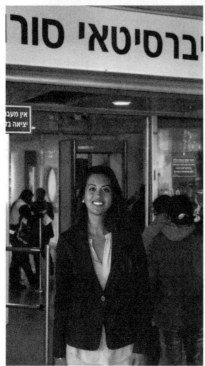

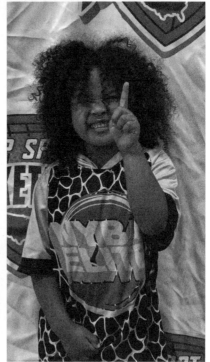

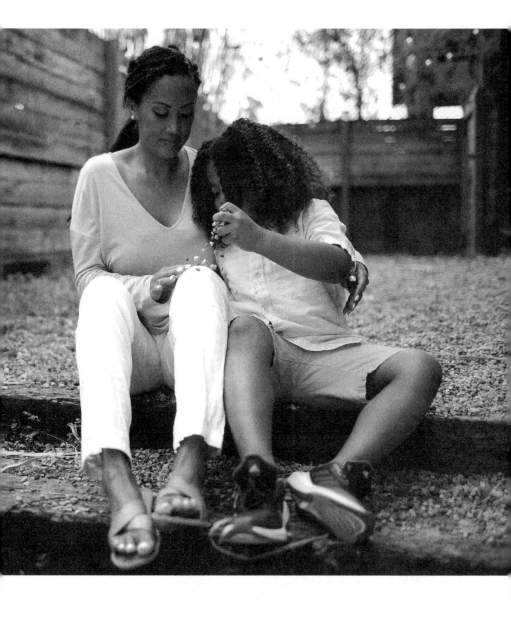

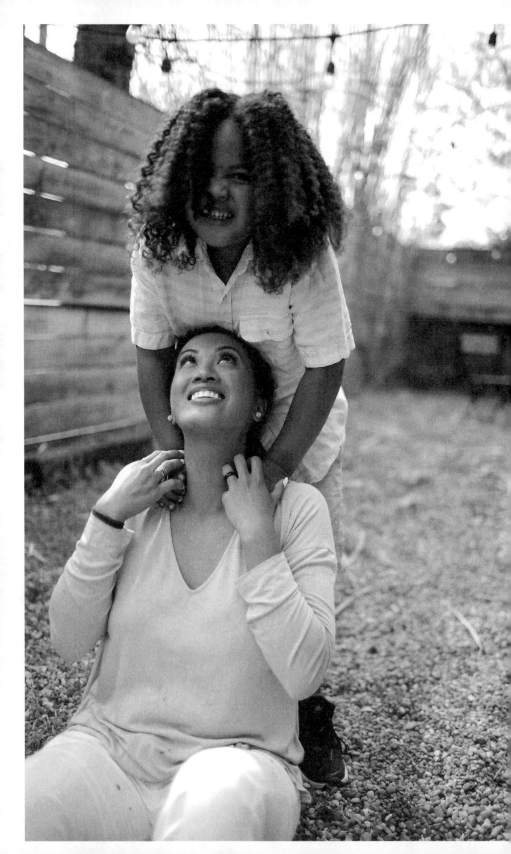

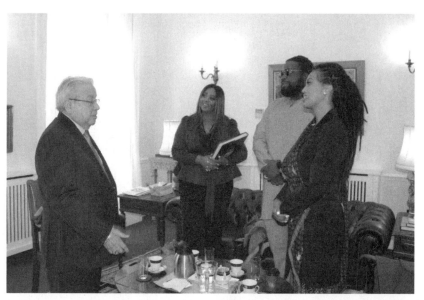

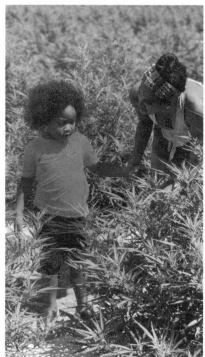

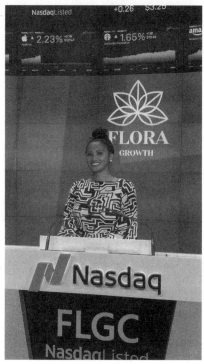

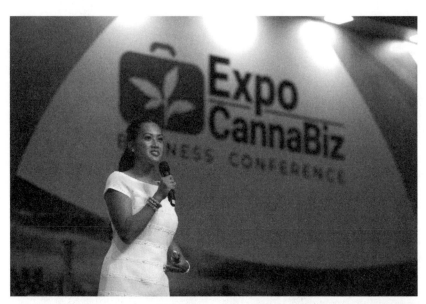

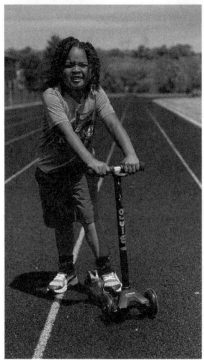

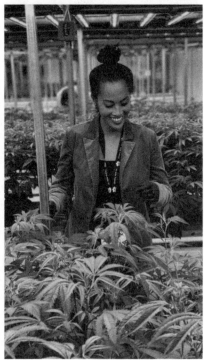

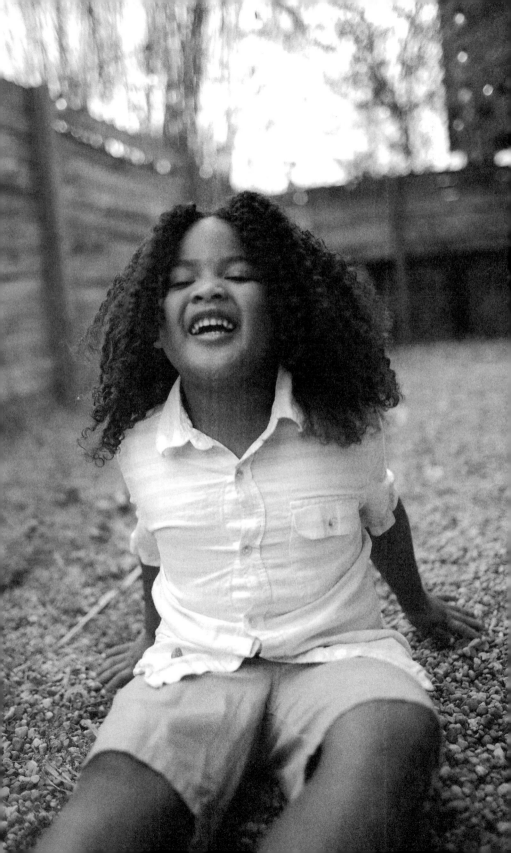

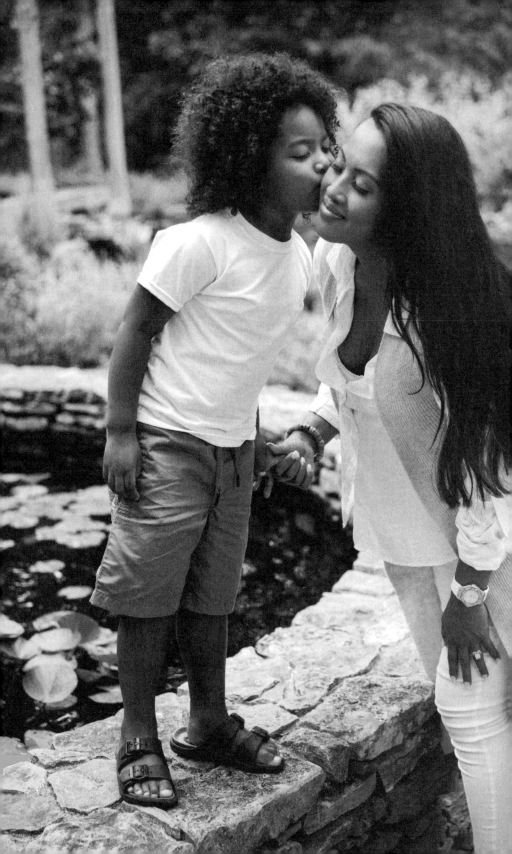

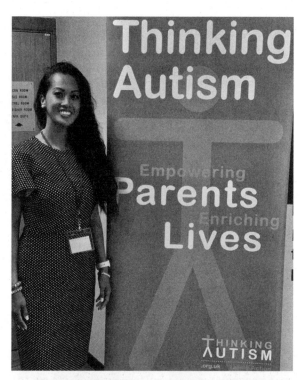

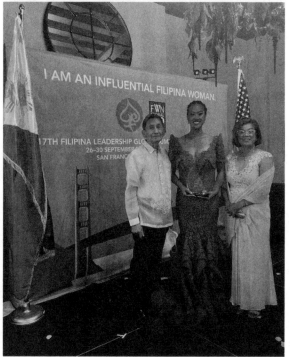

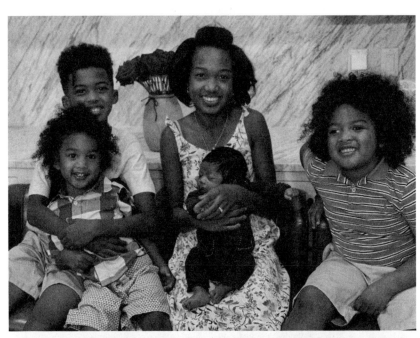

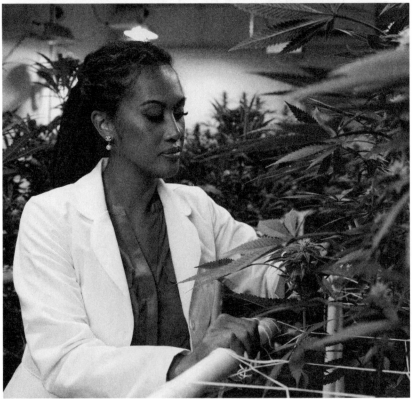

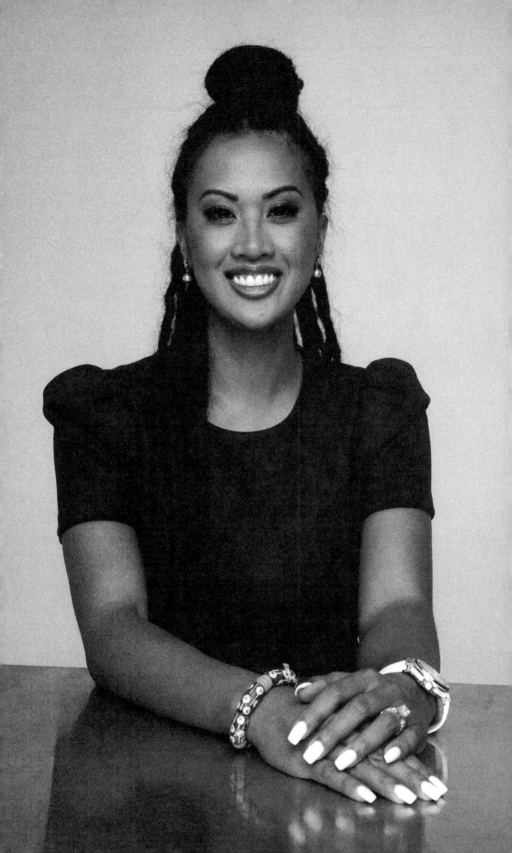

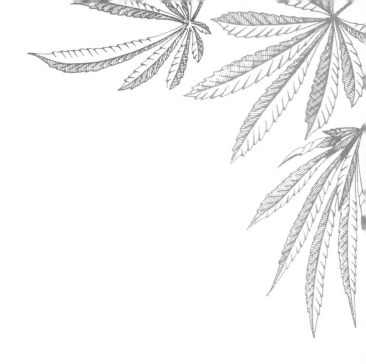

CHAPTER 7

IT'S ALL COMING TOGETHER

I f Macario's birth represents a fork in the road of my life's journey, his miraculous recovery represents a fork in the road of my professional destiny. Before Macario, I could never have predicted my entry into the cannabis research and development space. Now, I can't imagine my life outside of it. The process of developing a CBD oil and witnessing that product's impact on my own son in such a significant way provided the context for a new passion and a new journey. But as with any new path taken, it was not immediately obvious where that journey would lead.

I knew this path would be informed by where I came from—even a few months into Macario's recovery, I knew the years of training and experience that went into obtaining my PhD would not be in vain. I also knew this path necessitated spreading the word on all I had learned in those months. With a culture on the cusp of the CBD craze, it felt absolutely paramount to clarify this trendy cannabinoid's role in my son's epilepsy—but beyond that, I wasn't sure where best to lend my expertise and insights. In 2018, an article about Macario and my CBD oil was published in *Forbes*. It was personal yet informative, but I could not have predicted or expected the attention that came after its publication. From the emails I was receiving, it was clear there was a desire for more understanding and intellectual rigor around cannabidiol as well as cannabis more generally. It was also clear there was a market for more products. But I had no interest in cashing in on a trend. With the background of a scientist, the passion of a mother, and the thirst of a lifelong learner, I set off on a path that would ultimately take me around the world, meeting with global leaders to brainstorm about regulatory structures and cannabis futures, and taking a wide lens to the possibilities and potential cannabis research could offer to individual patients, to communities, to entire economies.

A SHIFT IN THE MARKET

Between the time I wrote the *Forbes* article and this book's publication, CBD exploded onto the marketplace. This overnight surge in popularity of a previously little-known substance has its origins in the 2018 Farm Bill, which effectively lifted the federal ban on hemp production by removing the plant from its Schedule I status under the Controlled Substances Act. According to the Farm Bill, hemp is defined[83] as a cannabis plant that contains no more than .3 percent of THC—any cannabis plant that contains more than this slight percentage is still classified as a Schedule I drug, on par, from a legal perspective, with heroin, LSD, and cocaine. While the bill introduces major gray areas in terms of research and state-by-state legality, the marketplace took immediate advantage of hemp's new status: THC may still be prohibited, but the nonpsychoactive cannabidiol looked ripe for a market entry. Aided in equal parts by celebrity testimonials (in 2019, Kim Kardashian hosted a CBD-themed baby shower), pop-science exclamations (Sanjay Gupta praised the benefits of CBD on *The Dr. Oz Show*), and media reports trying to analyze the CBD craze (the *New York Times* described it as a "voguish cannabis derivative"[84]), hemp-derived CBD products saw a 706 percent jump in sales from 2018 to 2019[85]—and the trend shows no sign of slowing.

Those CBD-infused products included oils and tinctures, but also lotions, candy bars, sports drinks, makeup ... you name it. Restaurants are adding CBD to their main courses, coffee shops are adding it to their lattes, even doughnut shops are cashing in and creating sweet concoctions bearing the CBD buzzword. CBD shows significant promise as a medicine—but that does not by any means suggest the products on the market today reflect that promise or anything at all outside of the acknowledgment of *CBD* as the latest consumer buzzword. The lack of consistency across products, not to mention lack of scientific rigor behind many of the claims found pasted to

---

83   John Hudak, "The farm bill, hemp legalization and the status of CBD: An explainer," Brookings, last updated December 14, 2018, https://www.brookings.edu/blog/fixgov/2018/12/14/the-farm-bill-hemp-and-cbd-explainer/.

84   Alex Williams, "Why is CBD everywhere?," *The New York Times*, October 27, 2018, https://www.nytimes.com/2018/10/27/style/cbd-benefits.html.

85   Danielle Kosecki, "What is CBD and why is it so popular right now?," CNET, last updated August 5, 2019, https://www.cnet.com/news/what-is-cbd/.

the back of tincture bottles and chocolate bars, directly correlates to the significant skepticism we see in the marketplace of ideas: we are not even two years into the CBD craze and media outlets are already portraying the cannabinoid as a fad, snake oil, and—as one marketing exec proclaimed—"the new avocado toast."[86]

CBD's newfound popularity only exposes the need for legitimization and research. The timing could not have been more perfect. As a formulator of a pure CBD oil, I could've followed a path toward financial success—but what would I have to show for it? To cash in on shoddy claims and questionable science is not an action my value system would allow me to take—not now, not ever. At the same time, I had to reckon with the fact that my formulation did indeed change the life of my son. Bodies and individuals are unique—what miracles can happen in one body may not translate to another's. I grappled with this on my own path, and the results demonstrated both the power of cannabidiol and the limitations of science.

WHAT WE KNOW, WHAT WE DON'T KNOW

As we've discussed at length in prior chapters, the cannabis space at this stage is mostly defined by what we don't know—we understand the baselines, but myriad unresolved questions leave the scientific community without answers to the full extent of cannabis's healing powers. Scientists have a working knowledge of THC and CBD, and much more research must be conducted for both in terms of their medicinal value. We know that in addition to these two cannabinoids, there are over one hundred additional cannabinoids found in the

---

86   Alex Williams, "Why is CBD everywhere?," *The New York Times*, October 27, 2018, https://www.nytimes.com/2018/10/27/style/cbd-benefits.html.

cannabis plant that we have not yet established scientific rigor around. That's over one hundred other possible healing salves, health remedies, prophylactics, and so much more that we can't possibly predict.

Beyond the cannabinoids themselves, we need a clearer understanding of the potential of the endocannabinoid system that processes them. We know the CB1 and CB2 receptors are part of the larger family of G protein coupled receptors, or GPCRs, which bind to extracellular substances and transmit their messages to intracellular molecules.[87] GPCRs and the messages and information they convey from external sources to inside the body's cell play a role in such a diversity of functions in our bodies that it is estimated up to 50 percent of prescription drugs on the market right now act by binding to these unique receptors.[88] Given that our cannabinoid receptors are a part of this family, what medicines could be developed that similarly target these receptors to bring results? In the brain, we know CB1 receptors are located on the ends of our central and peripheral nerves and can control neurotransmitter release, allowing for potent neuro-protectivity. How might we regulate this in the future? With high-expression areas of the brain responsible for movement, memory, and pain, how might we utilize these receptors in a selective and efficient manner? Beyond this, there are great clues to the endocannabinoid influence on pain circuitry, spasticity, antioxidant activity, and more. We know CB2 receptors can modulate the release of cytokines, which in turn influence inflammation. The future of medication for inflammation, pain, and so much more may lie in our ability to utilize our bodies' own mechanisms for creating and processing cannabinoids and endocannabinoids alike.

---

87   Kara Rogers, "G protein-coupled receptor," Britannica, accessed April 2020, https://www.britannica.com/science/G-protein-coupled-receptor.

88   "GPCR," Nature, accessed April 2020, https://www.nature.com/scitable/topicpage/gpcr-14047471/.

RECOGNIZING CBD'S POTENTIAL

Given the gaps in our knowledge, when I was approached by multiple parties to use my knowledge of CBD to develop lotions or on-trend products, I had to draw a hard line in the sand and said no. On a case-by-case basis, however, I felt compelled to share my CBD oil with friends and friends of friends who might benefit. Anecdotal evidence must always be taken with a grain of salt—and more studies are absolutely needed to elucidate the mechanism of action, the hows and whys, behind each success story—but if my experiences sharing CBD with my inner circle are proof of anything, they're proof of the promise of this cannabinoid—and proof that the cannabis plant deserves to be taken seriously as a medicine and not simply subjected to the market trends of a given era.

The cannabidiol formulation I created for Macario was non-specific. It was not designed to stop seizures or to heal a particular condition. Rather, it was formulated to regulate homeostasis. In some ways, our bodies are designed to heal themselves, and within our healing agency, the endocannabinoid system is a significant player. My CBD oil was designed to tap directly into that system—simply to awaken it is to direct its power in whatever way the body needs.

After I administered my product to Macario, I gave it to friends and acquaintances who were suffering from a range of maladies. One friend had fibromyalgia. He couldn't get out of bed. I gave him CBD and it helped, but not enough. Wanting to help, and armed with what working clinical knowledge I had, I designed a cannabinoid formula specific to his case—and now, he has no symptoms.

Another friend of mine suffered from type 1 diabetes. She's used long-term and short-term insulin since age twelve. She changed her diet and began to take CBD—and saw a significant balance in her sugar for the first time in decades.

My CBD oil helped a friend suffering from dystonia, it's helped autism in young children, and it's even caused multiple complete reversals in cancer patients. I'm so thankful to have played a role in healing these individuals and mitigating their pain—yet I recognize that it is not my place, in the long run, to play the role of a physician. Perhaps you can infer the reason why: I can't in good conscience give out a product outside of my inner circle that has not undergone significant clinical trials and passed the level or rigor that we require of all our medicines.

Do I believe in my own CBD oil? Of course. But I also recognize its limitations. For some people, CBD alone works wonders. But what works for one person may not work for another—and because my own formula has not gone through the rigorous trial phase I'd expect from other medications, I would not presume to establish my CBD oil at this stage as anything other than experimental.

> Do I believe in my own CBD oil? Of course. But I also recognize its limitations.

Ultimately, I don't believe my path was laid out for me to be a healer to specific individuals on a one-off basis. True impact is making change to the system itself—changing the way medicine is implemented so that I can help more than just the few that are able to see me. The anecdotal evidence is phenomenal, but understanding the mechanisms and pathways underlying each success story will allow me and other scientists and doctors alike to help not just a few individuals, but thousands—perhaps millions—over time.

And that's what I'm after, in the end. Systemic change, collaboration with partners across the world to make sense of what's right under our noses: the cannabis plant. The cannabinoids we know about, the cannabinoids we have yet to investigate, our endogenous cannabinoids and the mechanisms by which we process them. To successfully treat one individual is a blessing. To discover how we could treat hundreds of thousands with similar symptoms, whether from cancer, fibromyalgia, epilepsy, diabetes, or countless other possible illnesses, would be more than a blessing—it would be a completion of a life's work, my work, a completion of the path I was set on by the birth of Macario.

CANNABIS AROUND THE WORLD

I believe we are each blessed with certain gifts in life, gifts that our background, upbringing, and experiences hone over time—and one of the greatest blessings is to be able to utilize those gifts to the benefit of our greater community. Partly due to nature and partly due to nurture, I recognize my gifts for being an adaptable, resilient person, someone who is open to where life leads and never strays from a new connection. And I began to wonder: what connections might there already be in the cannabis space—and what connections are just waiting to be made by the right person? Just as we can't understand the whole body by looking at a single system, we can't understand the world of cannabis by focusing on what's happening in just one country. If I wanted to learn, contribute, connect, and ultimately join like-minded people in making real change, I knew I would have to start viewing the cannabis space with a more global lens. What do cannabis research, attitudes, and trends look like elsewhere in the world? What could we learn from other countries, and what might they learn from us?

The world is experiencing a global shift in attitudes toward cannabis, and my travels certainly underscored that evolution. Whereas just decades ago, cannabis was not only largely taboo but punishable by significant jail time, governments around the world are now moving to relax their laws on the plant. Like any major shift in beliefs or attitudes, there is no single factor that can be attributed as the root or primary cause, but rather a multiplicity of factors, trends, and incentives that have coalesced to move the dial toward legalization and general curiosity, and away from fear and punishment. First, the moral panic introduced in the early twentieth century is slowly but surely being disproven with every new cannabis study published. *Reefer Madness* would have the world believe cannabis makes people violent, is highly addictive and morally destructive, and has numerous other terrible impacts. Of course, none of those impacts panned out in the decades that followed. And in fact, the opposite has turned out to be true: not only is cannabis generally harmless, it has positive impacts on numerous health ailments, and as I've underscored throughout this book, we have so much more to learn. Second, cannabis is the most widely grown and used illicit drug on earth.[89] By legalizing its use, countries can help to curb its trade on the black market and bring some level of regulation to users. Third, the combination of these first two factors—its relative harmlessness and its relative ubiquity—makes the plant a potential economic behemoth, which states like Colorado[90] and countries like Canada are already capitalizing on to positive results.

Over the past five-plus years, I spoke to dozens of leaders and change-makers from all over the globe. My understanding of cannabis blossomed into something both powerful and rewarding, and my

---

89   "A global revolution in attitudes toward cannabis is under way," *The Economist*, last updated August 29, 2019, https://www.economist.com/international/2019/08/29/a-global-revolution-in-attitudes-towards-cannabis-is-under-way.

90   Mona Zhang, "Legal marijuana is a boon to the economy, finds study," *Forbes*, last updated March 13, 2018, https://www.forbes.com/sites/monazhang/2018/03/13/legal-marijuana-is-a-boon-to-the-economy-finds-study/.

insights only served to strengthen my belief that cannabis is the next frontier of medicine, if only we'd loosen our regulatory reins and evolve our remaining collective biases. What follows is a survey of some of the places I traveled and some brief takeaways that help shed light on the future of cannabis medicine.

ISRAEL

It could be fairly said that no single country has done as much for cannabis research as Israel. Not only was Israel one of the first countries in the world to legalize cannabis, it was here that both THC and CBD were first isolated from the cannabis plant—and, subsequently, it was here that the endocannabinoid system was first discovered. Much of the pioneering work can be traced back to one scientist's body of work in particular: that of Professor Raphael Mechoulam, of the Hebrew University in Jerusalem. As the story goes, in the early 1960s Mechoulam had a simple question: why was it that the active compounds from poppies and coca leaves (opium and cocaine, respectively) had long been isolated, studied, and exploited, and yet the cannabis plant remained a mystery?[91] Seeking to find out, Mechoulam obtained a sample of smuggled hashish from the local police and, with a team of collaborators, began to examine the substance. Their isolation of CBD and THC catapulted Mechoulam and his research team into fame and inspired generations of scientists to continue the exploration.[92] Tellingly, their work built off a body of research created by an American chemist named Roger Adams, whose efforts to study

---

91   Abbie Rosner, "Dr. Raphael Mechoulam, the Godfather of cannabinoid research," *MG Magazine*, July 17, 2019, https://www.cfhu.org/news/prof-raphael-mechoulam-hus-godfather-of-cannabinoid-research-spotlights-latest-work/.

92   Karin Kloosterman, "Israeli medicine goes to pot," ISRAEL 21c, last updated March 29, 2012, https://www.israel21c.org/israeli-medicine-goes-to-pot/.

the chemical components of cannabis were stifled by J. Edgar Hoover in the 1940s.[93]

Mechoulam's work raised a natural question: now that two specific cannabis compounds had been isolated, what, precisely, was the body's biological mechanism for processing those compounds? That mechanism was found by a US scientist named Allyn Howlett, who first discovered the existence of our CB1 and CB2 receptors in the mideighties. Of course, this discovery led to yet another pertinent question: surely these receptors don't exist in our body for the sole purpose of processing cannabinoids from external substances? Mechoulam evolved the body of research yet again in 1992 in his discovery of endogenous compounds that activate these receptors. He named the first compound he found "anandamide." *Ananda* in Sanskrit means "complete joy." Three decades later, Mechoulam, his peers, and many other prominent scientists have implicated the endocannabinoid system in essentially all human disease. The importance of this implication simply cannot be overstated.[94]

No doubt because of the legitimacy Mechoulam's research lent to the plant, cannabis has been taken seriously in Israel for decades—so seriously, in fact, that Yuval Landschaft, the pharmacist who leads the Israeli Health Ministry's Medical Cannabis Unit, frowns upon the use of *marijuana* versus *cannabis* in order to "avoid lingering stigma" and help to distinguish the medicinal value of the

93   Tracy Wilkinson et al., "Israel is banking on cannabis as its next big industry," *Los Angeles Times*, May 29, 2019, https://www.latimes.com/nation/la-fg-israel-cannabis-medical-marijuana-20190529-story.html.

94   Meir Bialer, "Raphael Mechoulam and the history of cannabis research," *ILAE Journal*, Epigraph Volume 21, Issue 1, Winter 2019, https://www.ilae.org/journals/epigraph/epigraph-vol-21-issue-1-winter-2019/raphael-mechoulam-and-the-history-of-cannabis-research.

plant from its recreational value.[95] Cannabis was first legalized for prescription use in 1973, and in 2019 the government voted in favor of permitting cannabis exportation. In Israel, regulations for clinical trials are more relaxed, so the entire process of cannabis drug development is significantly smoother. Recognizing the significant lack of research in the medical cannabis space and the legal constraints that prevent this problem from being addressed elsewhere in the world, Israel has even gone so far as to create a research and development committee comprised of experts in the life sciences, chemistry, medicine, and agricultural fields that meets quarterly to discuss pertinent issues.

This history of scientific and intellectual rigor set the context for my visits to Israel, where I had the pleasure of meeting some absolutely phenomenal scientists who continue to build on their strong foundation through both clinical trials and the publication of important research. And yet even this pioneering country has its challenges when it comes to cannabis. Right now, there are nearly fifty thousand patients in Israel who can receive medical cannabis for ailments ranging from epilepsy to obesity and many health concerns in between—but thousands more remain on the waiting list. During my travels, I had the opportunity to sit with a man in his eighties who had a long history of prescribing cannabis—he was the first doctor to prescribe cannabis to a patient with AIDS. He told me about the struggle some Israelis have faced in procuring cannabis, and how upsetting that is given how amazing the results have been. Israel may be the most established in the cannabis-as-medicine space, but in contemporary society it is not yet as readily accessible as it may seem.

95   Tracy Wilkinson et al., "Israel is banking on cannabis as its next big industry," *Los Angeles Times*, May 29, 2019, https://www.latimes.com/nation/la-fg-israel-cannabis-medical-marijuana-20190529-story.html.

Beyond accessibility issues, I had also expected to see more of a protocol when it came to the administration of medical cannabis. It is important to be able to collect data in this new area of science, and yet in this area, too, Israel seems to be on par with other countries where one might think it would be ahead. This all led me to one of my biggest takeaways: Israeli scientists may be at the forefront of their research, but they can't do it all alone. Cannabis is complicated and complex—in terms of medicine alone, it will take collaboration between other big players to make meaningful, long-lasting impact.

> Cannabis is complicated and complex—in terms of medicine alone, it will take collaboration between other big players to make meaningful, long-lasting impact.

CANADA

While Israel may be the pioneer of cannabis research, Canada—which legalized recreational cannabis in October 2018—is undoubtedly thought to be its next frontier. Cannabis use and regulation underwent a similar historical trajectory in Canada as it did in the United States, with vilification of the drug reaching a fever pitch in both countries by the late sixties. But there was one marked difference between the two geographies that helped to pave the way for cannabis's newly legal status in Canada. When cannabis use began to skyrocket in the sixties, the government responded in a pragmatic manner, with Prime Minister Pierre Elliott Trudeau—father of current Prime Minister Justin Trudeau—appointing a royal commission to learn more about cannabis's actual impacts on the health of the body and brain. Led by Gerald Le Dain, the commission commenced its study in 1969 and completed its work three years later. Its findings stated there was "zero science" to back criminal sanctions for marijuana possession, clarifying that the report did not mean to encourage the use of cannabis but rather to "reduce the impact of the criminal law."[96] In a particularly prescient moment, the report also recommended the federal government conduct additional research to evaluate long-term effects of cannabis.

Pierre Trudeau's government largely ignored the report, but its commissioning and publication were still significant. Fifty years later, and nearly two decades after medical cannabis was made legal, Trudeau's son finally took action by making Canada the first major economy in the world to legalize recreational cannabis.

The sale of cannabis has exploded in the last few years—but in my visits to Canada, I found a lack of direction on the medicinal side of things. Recreational cannabis and medicinal cannabis are simply not the same thing, and conflating them can lead to less-than-optimal results. In one case, I visited with a family who had high hopes a cannabis medication could help their autistic child. I looked at the product, and it was a dirty extract of cannabis with such a low dosage that it was almost certainly not going to have an impact—and it didn't.

As a native Canadian, I feel a personal stake in this: I want to see Canada producing good, clean cannabis medication that's transparent, consistent, and backed by studies. But as with other countries, Canada is struggling on the issue of research. Science takes time, and the way we have approached science with cannabis is in such a rushed manner. Almost as if there is a push from the recreational space in order to make new medicines and technologies. The root molecular science does not seem to get any attention, and it usually never does. The scientific community was understandably excited at the prospect

---

96   J.S. Bennett, "Le Dain Commission inquiry into the non-medicine use of drugs tables fourth and final report," *Canadian Medical Association Journal*, January 5, 1974; 110(1): 105–108, https://www.ncbi.nlm.nih.gov/pmc/articles/PMC1947221/.

of cannabis legalization and the research prospects it would open up. However, researchers still need a permit to study cannabis's medical uses, and the CBC has reported that significant bottlenecks in funding have occurred since legalization, leading to a lack of clinical trials. There have also been reports about lingering biases in the way government grants are being given to cannabis researchers. According to the Canadian Institutes of Health Research, there are three research streams that apply to cannabis: medical benefits, data standards, and understanding harms—but it's the latter that seems to be getting the most traction in terms of grant funding.[97]

Canada's legalization has only been in effect for a couple of years, and certainly many of its issues around research, funding, and developing medicines could be qualified as mere growing pains—pains that, once sorted, will hopefully lead to more fruitful results for both the research field and for patients more generally.

SOUTH KOREA

I was asked to go to South Korea with a good friend who was embedded in the current medical cannabis legalization process. In late 2018 South Korea became the first country in East Asia to legalize medical cannabis for specific ailments, a move that was recognized around the world as a significant turn from a decades-long policy of harsh punishment for cannabis users.[98] South Koreans can be penalized with up to five years in prison or a fine of over $40,000. Because of this, the

---

97   "Regulations, funding keep Canada from becoming world leader in cannabis research, scientists say," CBC, last updated October 19, 2019, https://www.cbc.ca/news/canada/manitoba/canada-cannabis-research-barriers-1.5326667.

98   Sintia Radu, "South Korea approves medical marijuana," US News and World Report, last updated December 12, 2018, https://www.usnews.com/news/best-countries/articles/2018-12-12/south-korea-is-the-first-east-asian-country-to-legalize-medical-cannabis.

number of drug arrests in the country is decisively small—in 2015, twelve thousand drug arrests were made in a population of over fifty million people.[99] Cannabis is still very much taboo in South Korea, to the point that it seems the entire country is afraid of the plant. There are very few advocates, but the few there are have a big vision and are working hard to change the mind of the government. South Korea prides itself on having a drug-free reputation, so they have a long way to go. But the small change in the law to allow certain prescription cannabis drugs is certainly a step in a more open and accepting direction.

Only a small number of cannabis drugs are approved in South Korea, and to obtain them patients must show their medical records as well as a physician's note clarifying there is no alternative. I am in weekly communication with my network in South Korea—and this will be one place to watch in the coming years as cannabis opinions continue to evolve from the taboo reputation to acceptance.

AUSTRALIA

Like South Korea, Australia remains on the conservative side when it comes to cannabis research and use. In 2016, the country's parliament passed legislation that allowed the cultivation of cannabis for certain medicinal and research purposes—including research on cannabis's impact on epilepsy, multiple sclerosis, chronic pain, chemotherapy, and HIV/AIDS—but otherwise cultivation remains illegal.[100] The govern-

---

99   Benjamin Haas, "Bong arm of the law: South Korea says it will arrest citizens who smoke weed in Canada," *The Guardian*, last updated October 23, 2018, https://www.theguardian.com/world/2018/oct/23/bong-arm-of-the-law-south-korea-says-it-will-arrest-citizens-who-smoke-weed-in-canada.

100   "Alcohol, tobacco and other drugs in Australia," Australian Institute of Health and Welfare, last updated January 21, 2020, https://www.aihw.gov.au/reports/phe/221/alcohol-tobacco-other-drugs-australia/contents/drug-types/cannabis.

ment currently only allows a few companies to grow the plant and is administering cannabis to patients at a ridiculous price. There does not seem to be any patient tracking or moves toward large-scale research.

I met my Australian team through a famous Australian shaman, and although my work there is early, I came to realize that people of all types just want what's best for everyone—but with too few advocates and a conservative-leaning government, decisions in this arena come very slowly.

AFRICA

There are myriad reasons for countries to legalize the sale and purchase of cannabis, ranging from the positive implications on access for scientific research to the economic benefits of introducing a lucrative crop to the market. Perhaps nowhere in the world is the latter truer than on the African continent, where some researchers project the legalization of cannabis could represent a seven billion dollar market by 2023.[101] The reason for this projection is twofold. First, with over 13 percent of its population using cannabis, Africa is both the world's biggest producer and the biggest consumer of the plant. Second, certain regions in Africa boast optimal growing conditions for cannabis, and communities have a strong history and expertise in agriculture that could aid in successful cultivation. For now, however, cannabis is legal in just three countries. In 2017, Lesotho became the first country in Africa to legalize the cultivation of cannabis for medicinal purposes; despite its illegal status before then, over 10 percent of the country's arable land was already being used by farmers to grow cannabis, and the plant made up over

---

101   Shoshana Kedem, "Africa's budding cannabis market," *African Business Magazine*, last updated July 10, 2018, https://africanbusinessmagazine.com/sectors/agriculture/africas-budding-cannabis-market/.

60 percent of crop-based revenues.[102] In April of 2018, Zimbabwe became the second country to legalize marijuana for medical and scientific use, and in September of that year, South Africa decriminalized the cultivation and use of cannabis for private consumption. As with the other countries listed above, legalization is such a new experiment that growing pains are as abundant as the possibilities for the market—and with more countries in Africa likely to follow suit, including Eswatini (formerly Swaziland) and Uganda, Africa is an important space to watch in the coming years as the opportunities grow.

When I first went to Africa, my eyes opened to the possibilities—in fact, it was here I saw more of a need for a variety of uses of hemp than any other place I'd seen. From its potential for growth on virgin soil to its potential to create countless jobs for people, cannabis has the power to make big change in these struggling countries. I believe it could even help to reverse the number of people faced with disease.

One individual I've spent a lot of time with now is Jerry Rawlings, the former president of Ghana and a man who has done many great things for both his people and for all of Africa. I met him through my husband's work in the country, and after learning of Rawlings's political leadership and dedication to the working class in his own country, who continue to hail him as a hero, I became deeply inspired by both the power and vision one man or woman can instill and by the positive team-building and collaboration that can occur around that power. Jerry listened to my story and became one of the strongest backers for the things I'm motivated to do in Africa, starting with Ghana.

---

102   Danielle Edwards, "Lesotho acts as gateway to African cannabis market," *Cannabis Investing News,* last updated November 11, 2019, https://investingnews.com/daily/cannabis-investing/lesotho-gateway-african-cannabis-market/.

Africa represents an entire continent of opportunity, but the pitfalls that could occur are dangerous and must be noted before the industry takes off. Most importantly, the infrastructure for a new cannabis economy must prioritize local workers and local economies. Eoin Keenan, a consultant at a European-based cannabis market consultancy called Prohibition Partners, put it best in a recent interview with *African Business Magazine*. He states that with African businesses playing catch-up in a global market, it's an "absolute necessity that legislators and regulators develop a framework to ensure that local governments and companies support, develop and encourage local producers and processors" in order to "create and promote local sustainable cannabis economies that aren't just monopolized or dominated by foreign interests."[103] Keenan calls it a "fine balancing act," and I agree—the future of the industry will depend on the ability to develop frameworks that work with both local communities and profit in mind.

THE BOTTOM LINE

No one individual can advance cannabis research or a cannabis product far enough along that it changes an industry. My decision to take my knowledge and bring it into the collaborative fold with global leaders transformed my perspective and deepened my understanding in ways that continue to ripple outward. Each country is on a different timeline with cannabis legalization,

> No one individual can advance cannabis research or a cannabis product far enough along that it changes an industry.

103 Shoshana Kedem, "Africa's budding cannabis market," *African Business Magazine*, last updated July 10, 2018, https://africanbusinessmagazine.com/sectors/agriculture/africas-budding-cannabis-market/.

regulation, and research. Some countries are grappling with logistical concerns like importation and exportation, while others are still evolving out of a conservative mindset that can at times seem like a holdover from decades past. It's hard to say which country is further ahead—a better and more important question is, who is doing the best research? In the end, that's the only question that will push us toward a brighter collective future. In the next chapter, I'll dig into the specifics of what my team and I are doing to contribute to that future—and I cannot underscore enough how grateful I am that my work has contributed to the global dialogue.

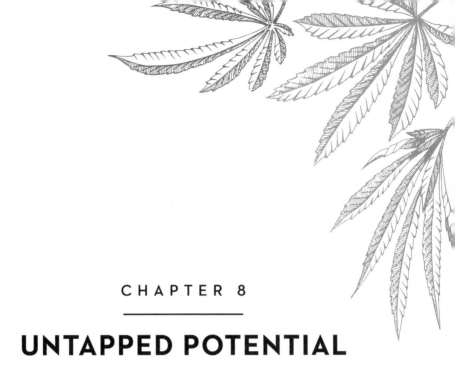

CHAPTER 8

UNTAPPED POTENTIAL

I n late 2019, I met with a friend in Washington, DC. My friend is a powerful, deeply admired woman in politics who has developed relationships with some serious game-changers over the last few decades. She also happened to be the first woman minority to receive a dispensary license in DC. During our conversation, she explained to me that there were limitations in the legalization, as medical dispensaries such as hers are only allowed to carry the cannabis flower—no tinctures, no capsules, no vaporizers, nothing else. At the end of the decade in 2019, in our nation's capital, the best we can offer medicinal cannabis patients is to toke up. My desire to see consistent and solid medicinal products is so far removed from our ability to look past cannabis as a psychoactive, smokable product. How can we bridge the gap from this moment to the future, where cannabinoids are accepted into our normal drug production line?

This book has taken you through the cultural and medical history of cannabis, the science behind how its molecules fit into our body's endocannabinoid system like a lock and key, and the myriad problems, biases, and taboos standing in the way of the research that could help harness the power of the plant and improve the lives of millions of patients. In the past hundred-plus pages, I have discussed the need for greater pathways of communication between scientist, doctor, and patient; the various cultural perceptions of cannabis; the pros and cons of various forms of administration and ingestion; and the global trends that are beginning to take shape in this burgeoning industry. As I've moved through these ideas, I've tried to underscore what this book is meant to provide: a broad philosophical and scientific overview of the cannabis plant and its game-changing potential. Cannabis has undergone sweeping pop-culture vilification for nearly one hundred years, and it's my hope this book has played a small role in debunking that harmful legacy and lending legitimacy to a plant that has been cultivated for its healing value for well over three thousand years.

I've also tried to underscore what this book is not meant to provide. I have not provided a detailed analysis of the medicinal attributes of cannabis, the precise mechanisms of action that make it work, or a rigorous list of ailments and the ways in which cannabis can cure them, because that analysis would simply be ethically irresponsible to offer at such an early stage in the research. I've pointed back to this ongoing theme in every chapter, if not every section: we have a mountain of evidence pointing to cannabis's potential. And we have almost nothing to show for how that potential should best be harnessed.

Unless we can back up promising claims with hard-won data and well-conducted studies, the cannabis industry is going to continue moving in circles, treading water until it sinks under the weight of its unfulfilled potential. Culturally, the industry's reputation will continue to rot with dubious claims, shoddy research, and useless products that leave the consumer skeptical that cannabis has anything of value to offer them, or is anything other than twenty-first century snake oil. Politically, the industry will remain a regulatory topic nobody wants to touch with a ten-foot pole. Medically, an entire generation of patients will suffer ailments that could've been made more bearable—*if only*. If only we took the time to put our money where our mouths are, if only we invested in the science, if only we stopped seeing the cannabis leaf primarily as a symbol of the subculture—if only we evolved our collective viewpoint and widened our cultural lens to contextualize our current historical moment. What would we find, if only we'd take a chance on this plant? And how many countless lives and communities would benefit?

My son's sickness was a low point of my life. In the hellish months between Macario's first seizure and his eventual recovery, one thought kept arising in the back of my mind: I would not wish my pain on any mother—and I would not wish Macario's pain on any child. I've said it before and I'll say it again: my CBD oil is not at a stage where I could feel confident administering it to patients as a direct answer for their ailments—nor does my degree or expertise warrant that. What works for one does not work for all; and yet, if cannabis does work for one, and to such transformational results, I believe the scientific community has a professional obligation to dig deeper. I know I certainly do.

I've outlined the whats, the what-ifs, and the whys of the future of cannabis as a plant, an industry, and a medical promise. In this chapter, it's time to move to the hows. In broad strokes, we know what that promising future will look like. I want to tell you what I am doing right now to get us there.

FILLING IN THE GAPS OF FUTURE CANNABIS MEDICINE

As of late 2019, over 90 percent of Americans believe medical cannabis should be legal. Nearly two-thirds believe cannabis should be legal for both medical and recreational use. And just 8 percent of the country believe cannabis should be illegal in all circumstances.[104] Slowly, our politicians are beginning to take note: just three major presidential candidates in the 2020 election oppose full federal legalization, but each of those three support states' rights to regulate. By the end of 2019, thirty-three states plus Washington, DC, had legalized cannabis in some form, and more than a dozen are pushing for legalization in 2020. In terms of the US market, cannabis sales are projected to grow by 25 percent in 2020, dramatically outpacing the prior year's sales of $13.6 billion.[105] Globally, the cannabis market is projected to grow by 32 percent, with sales increasing from just over $10 billion in 2018 to over $97 billion by 2026.[106] Change is coming to this industry whether we're ready for it or not—and that change is bringing in the type of revenue that could revolutionize this field. But where is that money going? We are at a make-or-break moment, right before the cannabis watershed, where leaders of the cannabis space can have a huge impact in shaping both cultural perceptions and the future of the industry—and we need to have a game plan.

---

104 Andrew Daniller, "Two-thirds of Americans support marijuana legalization," Pew Research, last updated November 14, 2019, https://www.pewresearch.org/fact-tank/2019/11/14/americans-support-marijuana-legalization/.

105 Kevin Murphy, "Greener growth for cannabis in 2020," Forbes, last updated December 26, 2019, https://www.forbes.com/sites/kevinmurphy/2019/12/26/greener-growth-for-cannabis-in-2020/#577e7d71136f.

106 Sweta Killa, "Cannabis ETFs are soaring in 2020: Will the trend continue?," Yahoo, last updated January 16, 2020, https://finance.yahoo.com/news/cannabis-etfs-soaring-2020-trend-155003310.html.

After years of traveling the world and speaking to these leaders, I've come up with a blueprint for the future that I think will steer us in the right direction for years to come. This blueprint is anchored in three core needs—current gaps in the industry—we must address: research, collaboration, and education. Below, I outline why each need is important and what I am personally doing to address it.

GAPS IN THE RESEARCH: WHAT'S MISSING AND WHAT WE'RE DOING ABOUT IT

Here's the hard truth about cannabis research: What the consumer wants and what the science requires are two different things. What people perceive as data and what scientists perceive as data are also two different things. It would be unfair and unrealistic to assume a lay consumer is familiar with the scientific process, but I do not think it is unfair for scientists to do a better job of explaining what that process is not. As just one example, claims are often made in the medical cannabis space that x, y, or z strain or product benefits x, y, or z ailment, and the only "studies" they have to back it up are anecdotal surveys where patients self-describe their experience. For numerous reasons, patient surveys are not reliable research, and when manufacturers or sellers market them as such, the credibility of the whole industry suffers.

To me, molecular studies, cell studies, and animal studies are the gold standard—and the more we have, the better. Molecular studies are about peeling back the onion and taking a very close look at how molecules work both alone and then together. These studies could help define and clarify not just the molecules of the cannabis plant— all one hundred twenty cannabinoids we currently know about, plus however many more we have yet to discover—but also how those molecules fit and operate within our own intercellular pathways. We are talking about defining the endocannabinoid system better, understanding what the normal patterning of cell signaling is, which biological players are involved, how endocannabinoids and exogenous cannabinoids have an impact on this system, and how this system subsequently has an impact on other bodily systems. These types of studies would help us understand the discrete mechanisms at play when CBD is added to a neuron-rich system like the brain, and how CBD might encourage those neurons to signal better—and that's just one example of many that we could understand better through the exacting lens of biology.

But right now, most of the money in the cannabis market is not going toward these studies—instead, it's going toward marketing and branding efforts, anything to sell a product. This is a short-sighted approach: what happens when the buyers of the product you're selling start to realize they're not getting what was advertised? Not only does your specific product lose a customer—the industry loses a supporter who might otherwise benefit from legitimate cannabis medicine.

If there's no universal standard, and if we know so little right now, and if government regulation only makes it harder for researchers to get answers... then what does cannabis science actually look like in practice?

All of this raises the question: if there's no universal standard, and if we know so little right now, and if government regulation only makes it harder for researchers to get answers … then what does cannabis science actually look like in practice? Right now, my team and I are working on three different studies and analyses that I hope will help to form the backbone of a body of work moving forward.

META DATA ANALYSIS

In an industry so full of noise, I believe the best place to start is to survey everything that's out there; filter out the false promises, the bad studies, and the incomplete work; and determine the value of what's left—and what's missing. That's exactly what we did with our meta data analysis. There are nearly twenty thousand papers on the subject of cannabis, and we are looking at every single one of them. Unfortunately, many of these studies were not peer reviewed, were not double blind, offered patient reports with flimsy controls and subjective outcomes, or had other obvious flaws that made them less than useful to the body of work as a whole. As we went through, I became very frustrated by how few studies made it through the sifting process—but this is important work, because now we have a starting point to clarify what is known, what is not known, and what needs more conclusive data.

With that starting point in mind, our team is conducting a second meta data analysis to survey what the body of literature says about individual known cannabinoids, whether or not they are applicable to a specific system and/or disease, and how they interact mechanistically both with the body and with each other. It also surveyed where the research stops on lesser-known cannabinoids—for instance, the cannabinoid cannabigerol, or CBG, is thought to have promise as perhaps the next CBD. Our analysis helped to clarify how much serious research bears this and other popular claims out—and how much more needs to be done before those claims move into the realm of observable science. This is exciting work that further focuses our attention and resources.

Another positive outcome from the meta data my team and I are collecting is the clarity it provides to which scientists are doing what and who might benefit from being connected to one another. One problem is people are studying cannabinoids and not necessarily knowing what to do with the results. They're discovering things that someone in my position, who has a big-picture view of the industry, can look at and contextualize into the wider web of knowledge being slowly created. It's tough for scientists to make connections without external help, because they get so focused on the hypothesis. Utilizing someone with a wider lens can lend greater clarity to where the research fits and how it can be furthered. This net good fits into my goal of better research as well as greater collaboration.

RIGOROUS STUDIES

Once the literature has been sorted and the gaps in the research have been quantified, we can begin to conduct molecular and cellular studies that aim to fill those gaps with high-quality research. In collaboration with teams in both the US and the Caribbean, my team's studies aim to build a foundation of knowledge for how endocannabinoid receptors are expressed, which are expressed in different cell times, and which phytocannabinoids interact with these cells and receptors. We also hope to determine how the environment of the cell is impacted. Much of this work will involve animal model and cell-based studies with individual cannabinoids targeting specific symptoms or diseases.

Other work we are conducting will focus on bioavailability and absorption rates. Delivery has always been a very strong concern of mine: who cares what you put in your mouth if it is not absorbed correctly? If you had the choice, wouldn't you want a pharmaceutical drug that has been shown to cross the blood–brain barrier with a swift absorption rate? When you take a Tylenol, you want it to work within minutes, not hours. And it does—because we know exactly how much Tylenol our body needs to absorb in order for the drug to work effectively within its specific target. The cannabis "medicine" on the market doesn't know what's being targeted, so we can't possibly know how much is needed. Our collaborative studies on bioavailability and absorption will provide crucial data to help ensure future medicine-grade cannabinoids are properly dosed and metabolized, feeding the endocannabinoid system in the most impactful way possible.

Research on the endocannabinoid system, on cannabinoids themselves, and on dosing, bioavailability, metabolization, and more are just the tip of the research iceberg. But I'm proud of what my team has been able to accomplish thus far in moving the ball forward—and there's more forward movement to come with every passing month.

COLLABORATION: WORKING TOGETHER TO MAKE BIG THINGS HAPPEN

In chapter 4, I discussed the Upstairs Downstairs effect and the significant lack of communication that slows down our progress toward cannabis medicine. But the lack of communication is not strictly a problem between doctors and scientists—it exists in nearly every arena in the cannabis space. There's a lack of communication between scientists and cannabis industry leaders, between scientists and politicians, and between scientists themselves. This communication breakdown has led to two significant problems that greater collaboration could easily address: product standardization and greater regulation.

THE PROBLEM WITH STANDARDIZATION

The cannabis industry is so young that there are not yet universal standards when it comes to testing. There is little to no data on the products on the market, and no standardized way to measure their efficacy or claims.[107] Instead of buckling down, we're just making assumptions—and yet collectively, we are at an awakening where people are hungry for the truth and want to know more. We've gotten away thus far with saying "yeah, there's science being done," because the industry, largely lacking the backing needed from the scientific community, doesn't know what real science looks like. In this intellectual vacuum, big headlines fill the void and can shift perceptions on a whim.

> The cannabis industry is so young that there are not yet universal standards when it comes to testing. There is little to no data on the products on the market, and no standardized way to measure their efficacy or claims.

With more scientific studies and greater collaboration between lab and industry, we can begin to understand how specific products work within our bodies, and we can create and implement standards for those products to ensure both safety and efficacy. With time, effort, and communication, we can work together to ensure the market isn't selling useless CBD products that our bodies can't process. Like a ripple effect, good studies beget standardization and standardization begets good data: once we have clear universal standards, we can

---

107   Nick Jikomes et al., "The cannabinoid content of legal cannabis in Washington state varies systematically across testing facilities and popular consumer products," *Science Reports*, 8, 4519, 2018, https://www.nature.com/articles/s41598-018-22755-2.

implement real patient tracking systems and controlled trials. It's a virtuous cycle of knowledge.

The goal is simple: I want the market to match the evidence. I want to ensure people taking CBD, THC, or any other cannabis medicine actually benefit from the products they're buying. It doesn't have to be so complicated—collaboration between scientists and the industry would help.

THE PROBLEM WITH REGULATION— OR THE LACK THEREOF

Medical cannabis dispensaries are open in more states than not—and more and more are opening around the globe. Troublingly, because of the lack of science and standardization, there are no clear regulations in place ensuring product safety and transparency. Imagine this scenario: An elderly woman goes into a dispensary to purchase something to help her with her pain and memory. She tries it and it works! Now, say she wants to buy it again, months later. There is no guarantee her repeat purchase will have the same result. Why? Because we don't know why the result occurred in the first place—products have so much variability that cannabinoid composition changes from bottle to bottle, and we have no regulations over what's in each product that would ensure its molecular replication. This is medical insanity—and it can't stand for long.

We collectively crave definition and transparency in our products—the current recreational market hinges on the characterization of indica vs. sativa strains, because we know what kind of high we want. And yet this dichotomy represents a huge overgeneralization of cannabis, which is far more complex than just these two categories. If we had clearer definition of which compounds did what, we could build out a more robust system of categorization, and we could regulate the products in each category to ensure they're working as advertised. By prioritizing transparency, the elderly woman buying cannabis for her pain could be guaranteed her repeat purchases each had the same biochemical makeup—no filler, just medicine.

A COLLABORATIVE FUTURE IS INEVITABLE— BUT WE NEED HELP GETTING THERE

Someday, I believe we will collectively look back on these days as the Wild West of the cannabis industry. I do believe strongly there will come a time when standardization and regulation will fall into place—but in order to get us there, we need to create the foundation to support the eventual build-out of both. In the spirit of collaboration and knowledge sharing, I am communicating with politicians, scientists, and doctors both in the states and around the world to get a general understanding of the myriad pathways toward legalization and the pitfalls standing in the way. I'm reading various bills and getting to know the state-by-state differences in perspectives. I'm attempting to get the right lawmakers in charge so that we can have some form of regulation—because once that's done, the science will fall appropriately in line. Like meta data analyses are needed before we can dive into specifics, so, too, is this big-picture view warranted before we can set out a plan to tighten the reins on the medical cannabis industry and get it moving toward a place of legitimacy and depth.

My team and I are also supporting companies and groups that are willing to do things the right way. Standardization and regulation are dual needs that are intricately intertwined: it's hard to have one without the other. In the push for a more consistent product, I am consulting on clinical trial designs and product development and encouraging relevant parties to ensure patient data is being collected. And in the push to regulate those products, I am working with specific states and countries to legalize cannabis in a way that prioritizes the patient and not the business.

Right now, there is nobody tying all the pieces of the cannabis puzzle together. Now and into the future, my goal is to use every connection I have to do just that: to highlight great research, to put people in touch, to get the right people grants, and to help evolve the many disparate players into an interconnected community all focused on the same goal: cannabis medicine that we can be proud of and that patients can both access and trust.

Ultimately, everyone in the cannabis space has a role and nobody can do it all themselves—but if we work together, we are dangerous.

A PROPER EDUCATION

In a sense, you can think of these three goals—research, collaboration, and education—as ever broadening circles of influence. If specific research goals benefit the scientists working toward them, and collaboration benefits both scientists and other thought leaders in other relevant categories looking to rein in a bucking medical market, then proper education benefits all of the rest of us—the culture writ large, the generational zeitgeist we all work to build and perpetuate. As the science progresses and lines of communication lead to standardization and regulation, educating people on the power of the cannabis plant will become increasingly required across disciplines.

Cannabis education and understanding began nearly two hundred years ago with William O'Shaughnessy's writings on the plant—but vilification and moral outrage cut that legacy short, and there's been no continuation. There's no platform right now for cannabis education, and as a result, people are misunderstanding the shape cannabis is taking as a potentially revolutionary medicine. It's time to build the platform and push O'Shaughnessy's legacy forward.

My goal on the education front is simply to provide the truth of what we know. I am conducting lunch and learns, doing webinars with pharmacy groups and medical schools, and creating a continuing education course about cannabinoids as medicine with pharmacy associations and academic institutions. With regard to the latter, I have asked separate scientists and doctors to lend their expertise. There isn't much happening in the cannabis space in regard to education, science, and medicine, and so this class is meant only as a baseline or starting point.

Even the best providers are using the statement "we need more research" without putting a foot forward to do it themselves. I understand why: research takes funding, and making medicine is both expensive and time consuming. But if we put energy and money into filling the education gap, the potential of cannabis may be more easily unlocked. The reason for this is simple: simply educating someone has a domino effect on the connections they make and the influence they have. An educated person has the power to educate others, creating a dynamic community of people who may be willing to commit themselves to join this industry in a positive way. My work is a part of that influence, and so is this book. The more you know, the more we all know: knowledge spirals outward and lifts us all up.

A FUTURE FOR A MIGHTY FLOWER

When it comes to medical cannabis, iterating toward the future we want is going to take a lot of time and a lot of work. It's not as simple as saying "just legalize it," because even if cannabis is legalized, it doesn't necessarily mean patients know what to use or how to use it in times of sickness or ill health. Your doctor likely doesn't even know. Legalization might mean easier utilization, but patients are utilizing it by chance. Cannabis has had a long historical arc as a medicine. It's time we bring that arc into the twenty-first century and bend it upward toward greater, more precise, more effective medical outcomes. There are holes in the cannabis industry, and I aim to fill them. Pushing for better research, more collaboration, and more robust education is where I choose to start.

My mission and my passion is to influence the medicinal aspect of the plant: to pull together science, data from active users, perspectives from doctors and scientists, and other disparate threads and begin to weave them together to form a realistic view of where we are and where we need to go. We have the tools at our fingertips to redefine the future of cannabis medicine—and cannabis medicine in turn has the power to redefine the future of medicine writ large.

It is my belief that by paying attention to the points outlined in this chapter, we can convince scientists of the value of this research, we can convince legislators to regulate appropriately, and we can convince nonbelievers of the legitimacy of a plant that's been assailed for the last hundred years. We can bolster transparency in a confusing industry, we can pinpoint specific cannabinoids for specific conditions, and we can connect the dots between the science and medical use. This industry can be standardized, regulated, and honest. It can be of value to millions.

Cannabis right now is pure untapped potential—but it could be a promise. It's time we water the seed of this mighty flower and watch where it may grow.

> **It's time we water the seed of this mighty flower and watch where it may grow.**

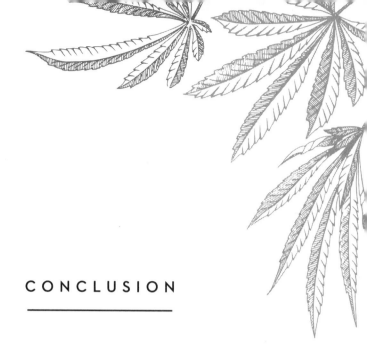

CONCLUSION

Sometimes you just have to marvel at life's timing. When things are going as planned, we allow ourselves the illusion of control over our lives. When the sea is calm, we feel we are the captains of our own ship. We forget that we are at the mercy of the waves—and that when a storm eventually hits, all we can do is try to stay afloat. There are certain moments in life—victories, tragedies, and other curveballs—that serve as vivid reminders that there are forces far bigger at play in the universe that we cannot understand and certainly cannot control. I call it God, but call it fate, call it the butterfly effect or random chance—these forces exist, whether we like it or not.

These moments and what we do with them come to define the shape of our lives and our identities. Of course, if you're reading this conclusion, you already know how I feel about riding out the unexpected waves. I've done it my whole life, from my interrupted basketball career to the months when my dad got sick to the moment we knew

Macario's only chance in life would require the removal of nearly half his brain. Being able to adapt to what's out of my control, and even grow from it, has been a constant strength in my life, but here's the thing: when things are going well, even I can forget I'm not fully in charge.

In 2016, my life was changed by Macario's seizures. By mid-2017, I was able to walk into Macario's doctor's office and let them know that, thanks to the CBD oil I'd developed, I had successfully taken my son off every single prescription drug he'd otherwise have been taking for years to come. Macario was developing in ways everyone thought would be impossible—and it was only after we quit the pharmaceuticals cold turkey that any of his progress occurred. My family and I had been dealt a tragic hand, and we not only recovered from it, we were thriving, and my heart was full of the potential and promise of the substance that had made it possible. The next five years, my life changed significantly. I shifted away from a career in the lab to a career as a cultivator of leaders, a team builder, a collaborator, a speaker, a researcher, and an advocate. I'd never worked harder, and had never been more hopeful about what that hard work was going toward. Our knowledge and understanding of cannabis used to seem more akin to a block of ice floating in the sea. Now, to more and more individuals—leaders and laypeople alike—cannabis is an entire iceberg, and we're just beginning to discover its breadth.

Cannabis is an entire iceberg, and we're just beginning to discover its breadth.

I was writing this book in 2019, and by December I was nearing its completion. With a big vision for the new decade, I felt in control of the ship like never before. Then, a wave struck. I wasn't ready for it. But in its timing, I had to recognize life was giving me important lessons, and I needed to take note.

On December 30, 2019, I was lying next to Macario as he slept when suddenly I noticed his body was seizing. It lasted a minute and a half before he went right back to sleep. It was the first seizure he'd had, to our knowledge, since his surgery at five weeks old. I spent the whole night in the emergency room with Macario. My experiences during the course of our stay served as a harsh but absolutely necessary reminder that life is a process, and progress is never a straight line. What can you do when a problem you thought you resolved evolves into a new problem you must solve except be honest and humble about the journey?

My experiences also underscored the purpose of my work and my mission. In an almost uncanny way, sitting through that sleepless evening and talking to the neurosurgeon mirrored many of the ideas I've touched upon in this book, from the unnecessary stigma of CBD to the problems the Upstairs Downstairs effect presents.

When Macario's seizure struck, I felt the immediate guilt of a mother. Could I have done something differently? Should I have continued him on the CBD for longer? The moment brought me back down to earth—how could I go around healing others when my own son was stuck in the ER? After I told our doctors in 2017 that we'd chosen to take Macario off his medication and pursue an alternative route, the neurology team told us point-blank we didn't need them anymore. Cannabis is still spoken of in hospital wings as if it's forbidden and banned—and because of that, we have not had access to the typical follow-ups he should be getting from a neurology team. He should've had MRIs, follow-up EEGs. But because we made a decision outside of the current medical framework, we didn't have access. Between 2017 and Macario's seizure, we had not even set foot in a hospital. Now that we were back, I was adamant about working with the team to find answers for why we were here at all.

The team had our charts. They could easily access everything about Macario's medical history—the resection of part of his brain, the fact that months later we took him off all prescription meds to administer CBD instead. The kid they thought would never talk or speak had walked right into their offices that night singing to Elmo and playing on his iPad—Macario's life is a miracle, and yet the team displayed no curiosity and asked zero questions about how the hell this had happened. There was no "tell me a little more about that," no "what specifically did you give him and are you still using it?"—nothing. The doctors should've sat there and said, "Given his history, we want to take a closer look." Instead, they just proceeded with the protocol they give every other child who comes into the ER after a seizure.

I could've told the team right then about my PhD in cell biology and background in developmental neuroscience, and what my suggestions would be in terms of tests I would run. Instead, I just listened to the doctors and asked questions as a concerned parent. I had a conversation with the doctor late at night, and he suggested we give Macario a one-hour EEG. An EEG picks up your brainwaves and can locate where a seizure occurs, when it occurs. Macario was hooked up to the EEG electrodes 24/7 all the way up to his surgery—and they wanted to do a simple, one-hour test. What's one hour going to pick up if he doesn't have a seizure within that hour?

I wanted a full MRI to determine what was happening. The doctor had a different idea. He told me it would be two to four weeks before my kid could get a brain scan. In the meantime, he said, "We're going to put him on Keppra." He explained this was the standard they start every child on when they are suffering from seizures. Keppra just so happens to be an extremely addictive, toxic medication that's not only hard to wean off but also has been shown to harm the development of the brain. It also just so happens to be the exact same drug

Macario had been on in the months following his surgery—one of the drugs I'd developed my CBD oil specifically to replace. Even aside from the problems Keppra introduced, this plan made no sense to me. We needed to know what was happening in the brain before medication. Doesn't waiting for a pill to normalize the brain and disrupt the seizure waves defeat the entire purpose of the scan? Why wouldn't we want to see what was working now so we could figure out the best personalized solution for my kid? It's like we were paving the way for him to stay on a harmful drug that at best should be used as a last resort, once all other options have been exhausted.

As I listened to the doctor explain his proposal for next steps, I realized just how distant the reality I'd been chasing was from the standard protocols. I'd spent the last three years of my life in an expansive space of discovery. In the search for a brighter future for my son, I'd grown so sure of the direction things were heading that I forgot how far we are from actually achieving them. My work doesn't look back—it looks forward, toward the potential of precision medicine, of cannabis medicine, of translational biology and an increasing dialogue between holistic care and modern treatment. My collaborators and I have spent years not just thinking outside the box of our healthcare system but trying our best to redefine what that box should look like as we move further into the twenty-first century. As I sat there in the ER, the box collapsed

> My work doesn't look back—it looks forward, toward the potential of precision medicine, of cannabis medicine, of translational biology and an increasing dialogue between holistic care and modern treatment.

in on me. If they'd wanted to, they could've given my son a brain scan within an hour. Instead, over seven hours of waiting later, and a thousand-dollar-plus bill growing by the minute, the doctor was presenting Keppra and a long wait for an MRI as the only option. I knew it was time to speak up when I had to hold back the urge to yell, "Do you know that I know what Keppra can do to my child?"

When I explained to the doctor my scientific background, his tone completely switched, and he told me they'd try to get Macario in for a brain scan as soon as possible. He even apologized for "dumbing things down." It's not that they were dumbed down, I wanted to say: you're just following a protocol that has no room for nuance. You're taking a medical concern comprised of a million different shades of gray and pretending it's black and white. That's not how bodies work. It's not how good health works. And I'm fed up with our healthcare culture behaving as though it is.

As I retell this story, it's hard not to feel cynical about the medical industry. Why was it that as soon as I told them of my background, I received a different, more personal treatment? My boy is going to be fine—but what about other kids and their parents who are in this same situation, who would've walked in there that day and walked out with a prescription for a serious drug and no explanation whatsoever as to the whats, hows, whys, and how longs about either the seizure or the drug itself?

I am hurt, mad, and worried all at the same time. Medical scares make us all vulnerable, and people deserve to be treated the same. I don't want to be treated like a customer in a bank line. I want to be treated like your friend, your family, like a person who is genetically different from every other person on this earth and needs personalized care—because we are, and we do. If I'm entrusting my family's well-being to you, I want to feel like you actually care that we're well in the first place. It's this business-as-usual approach, this adherence to inflexible protocols, and this lack of curiosity about both harms and alternative approaches that gave us the opioid epidemic. And it's not the doctors' fault. It's what is required of them, it's what our system has become. It bothers me that nobody wanted to know how CBD had helped my son—and it bothers me that despite CBD's explosion into the popular consciousness, we have not advanced even a little bit medically, and doctors' opinions remain as skeptical as ever. What happened to us in the emergency room that night is so indicative of everything that's wrong with healthcare today and of the frustrating pace of change in the industry. The only silver lining to our visit was that it verified every problem I've been working to address.

Ultimately, a kid missing 40 percent of his brain is liable to suffer complications. At his age, the brain is undergoing a transformational development—and there's only so much compensating that can be done before it hits a glitch. I'm putting Macario back on a heavy dosage of CBD moving forward and ordering tests to find out more. CBD replenishes systems and revitalizes signaling. It saved Macario once, and I have every confidence it'll restore his systems again. Keppra is a Band-Aid. Does it stop seizures? Yes. But I know what else it does to brain development, and if I can avoid it, I'm going to. We have so much more to learn and observe, and Keppra is not an option for us until we're sure all other options have been exhausted.

* * *

So where does that leave us? I'm not done with this journey—far from it. The work is incomplete. There's more to learn and more to accomplish. Life is fragile and imperfect, and my son's seizure was a reminder of the way we all must sit with the uncertainties and ambiguities it presents. I'll continue my work both in the United States and abroad, and when I come home, I'll look into my son's face and pray I am doing right by him and that he can always continue to smile and play like he can today.

Macario means blessing, and he's blessed our family beyond belief in ways I could've never planned for or predicted. I'm on this mission because of him—and because of him, I believe we're on our way to helping millions of lives with the cannabis plant. May his blessing continue.